ENVIRONMENTAL QUALITY AND ECONOMIC GROWTH

The Council of State Planning Agencies is a membership organization comprised of the planning and policy staff of the nation's governors. Through its Washington office, the Council provides assistance to individual states on a wide spectrum of policy matters. The Council also performs policy and technical research on both state and national issues. The Council was formed in 1966; it became affiliated with The National Governors' Association in 1975.

In addition to *Studies in Renewable Resource Policy,* the Council publishes:

■ *Studies in State Development Policy.* Current volumes include: *State Taxation and Economic Development, Economic Development: The Challenge of the 1980's, Innovations in Development Finance, The Working Poor: Toward a State Agenda, Inflation and Unemployment: Surviving the 1980s, Democratizing the Development Process, Venture Capital and Urban Development, Development Politics: Private Development and the Public Interest,* and *The Capital Budget.* Forthcoming volumes will address: the investment of public pension assets, banking and small business finance, state and local economic development strategies, the urban impact of federal policies, tax incentives, development finance theory, business taxation, and other topics.

■ *CSPA Working Papers.* Current volumes address: environmental protection and economic development; commercial bank financing for small business enterprise; the investment of public pension funds; the operation of minority capital markets; and the public service costs of alternative development patterns. A full list of current volumes is available on request.

■ *State Planning Issues.* A journal concerning the problems and practice of planning in the states. Published twice yearly.

■ *The State Planning Series.* Sixteen short papers dealing with financial management, citizen participation, econometrics, urban and rural development, policy development techniques, multi-state organizations, federal-state partnerships, and other issues of concern to state officials.

The Council of State Planning Agencies
Hall of the States
400 North Capitol Street
Washington, D.C. 20001
(202) 624-5386

Robert N. Wise
Director

Michael Barker
Director of Policy Studies

ENVIRONMENTAL QUALITY AND ECONOMIC GROWTH

ROBERT HAMRIN

STUDIES IN RENEWABLE RESOURCE POLICY

MICHAEL BARKER, GENERAL EDITOR

Copyright © 1981 by The Council of State Planning Agencies, Hall of the States, 400 North Capitol Street, Washington, D.C. 20001.

Library of Congress Catalog Number: 81-67187

ISBN: 0-934842-51-5

Printed in the United States of America. First Printing 1981.

Design: Kathy Jungjohann

STUDIES IN RENEWABLE RESOURCE POLICY

In the late 1960s and early 1970s, there was a great deal of passionate discussion about "the limits to growth," the collapse of the world's food system, the death of the oceans. To many Americans, the choices with which we were then being presented seemed unrealistic and harsh. The latter part of the decade featured adjusted models—less fearsome simulations—and the world continued to muddle along.

Unnoticed by many has been the emergence of several of the changes demanded by yesterday's prophets of doom. Although still embryonic, renewable energy sources are given increasing support, forest product companies discuss sustained yield harvesting, and resource recovery and recycling come and go in the public eye. Even the Bureau of Land Management now supports sustainable levels of grazing on public lands. In short, we are better prepared, both conceptually and analytically, to build bridges to an economy that is sustainable on a long-term basis.

In the long run, we are certain to consume all of our nonrenewable sources of energy and materials. A choice must therefore be made between the production and consumption of nonrenewables today, and their conservation for tomorrow. It is an important question of intergenerational equity. As things now stand, the economic choices of a very few generations can decisively influence the production and consumption abilities of all future generations. These limits apply not only to energy, which currently dominates public debate, but to the rate and way in which we use land (be it wilderness, forests, or agricultural lands) and the products of the seas. For some of these, we can ensure that no future generation can use a resource, as in the daming of Hells Canyon. For others, we may simply remove a resource for several generations, as in the excessive salting of overirrigated farmland.

One way of responding to this choice is to move towards an economy which produces and consumes material and energy at a rate and with a mix that is sustainable indefinitely. Such an economy would be based on resources known to be renewable (with proper management) despite their consistent use. In such an economy, nonrenewable resources would be used only until substitutes were found and made available for general use.

As already pointed out, we now have bits and pieces of this kind of

economy. Against great odds—energy pricing, regulation, a lack of capital—renewable energy is making its bid through small scale dams, photovoltaic cells, and other, now familiar devices. But a fully renewable economy would go further by encompassing the material requirements for overall production.

If we are to encourage the development of our economy in such directions, we must first pursue several underlying questions.

■　What would a renewable agricultural sector look like if called on to produce yields in a way that preserved the productivity of the land?

■　Do we have enough land to sustain a shift to natural fibers—such as cotton and wool—for most of our clothing needs?

■　What would be the approximate mix of feed grains, meat production, and biomass production for renewable energy if we came to rely on the sustainable capacity of the land rather than nonrenewable oil for fertilizers and much of our clothing?

■　What goods could we make out of wood? What level of sustainable yield would good management practices allow in the nation's forests? And what tradeoffs must we make with our desire to maintain certain wilderness areas in perpetuity?

■　How far can we go with the continuous recycling of the current stock of primary metals, such as iron, steel and aluminum?

■　What is the maximum sustainable yield on coastal fishing, and how far might it be augmented by aquaculture?

These are primarily technical questions. But while serious, they beg questions which are more serious still. How must our political and economic institutions change to permit a sustainable economy? What would be the impact of such an economy on the operation of markets and the allocation of income? What are the geographical implications of such an economy? Are states—or regions—an appropriate starting point for moving in such directions? Would interstate trade increase or decrease? What would happen if some states chose to move toward a more sustainable economy while others did not? And what can states— or individual local communities—do in the desired context of a market economy? What would some of the early transformations resulting from the movement to a more sustainable economy mean for the number and quality of jobs? the distribution of income? or the stability of local economies?

The past decade has produced a significant amount of literature relevant to these questions. Taken together, it is both analytical and quantitative, and political and moral. Although little of it was developed with precisely these questions in mind, we know far more than we did a decade ago about renewable energy, mineral reserves, and agricultural yields.

The purpose of this series is to clarify the boundaries and substance of this literature, to combine it with some clear conceptual thinking, and to extend it through an ongoing discussion and debate over the changes which must take place—in our policies, our politics, our public institutions—if we are to permit and encourage the emergence and growth of a sustainable, renewable economy.

Michael Barker,
General Editor

TABLE OF CONTENTS

INTRODUCTION

In the 1970s, the nation turned itself in a new direction. A commitment to environmental restoration was made and was backed by the enactment of some 20 major environmental statutes at the federal level alone. Perhaps no other problem with which we wrestled was as pervasive as that posed by the deterioration of our environment, or required such sudden, fundamental changes in both personal and corporate behavior. This redirection, comparable to the civil rights upheaval of the 1960s, has enriched the lives of all Americans.

Yet, it has not taken place without a considerable degree of controversy. In the first half of the 1970s, environmentalists charged that economic growth inevitably brings environmental harm and thus must be drastically reduced or even halted. The latter half of the decade was largely characterized by a counterattack, with business leaders in particular assailing environmental regulations as a major contribution to the country's economic woes.

This mutual suspicion and antagonism must cease if we are to surmount the large and complex challenges each field will present in the 1980s. A useful starting point would be a belated recognition that both "economics" and "ecology" share the same root, "eco"—derived from the Greek word for house or home. Thus, ecology is the study of the natural mechanisms of resource dynamics (or nature's housekeeping), and economics is the study of the human process of managing resources (or human housekeeping).

Beyond this, it is now time to explicitly acknowledge that economic growth need not in and of itself cause pollution, nor must environmental protection measures necessarily limit growth. The zero-sum mentality—economic growth vs. the environment—must give way to a recognition that the two are not only mutually compatible, but complementary in many ways. The environmentalism implicit in finding new and better ways to use and conserve energy is necessary for future economic growth. The economic growth achievable through the production and installation of pollution control equipment is key to environmentalism. Simply put, environmental values *are* economic values.

While such generalized abstractions *sound* good, it can be fairly asked what evidence there is to back them up. The five essays in this volume are meant to provide some preliminary evidence on the crucial

connections between economic and environmental trends and principles.

Briefly, the essays explore:

■ The ways in which environmental quality and economic growth can be brought into a positive, dynamic partnership

■ The economic incentives already at work in environmental regulations (the emission offset market and the bubble concept) as well as the often proposed emission charges approach

■ The neglect of natural resources and the environment, both in economic theory and policymaking

■ The argument that economic policies must be examined not only with respect to their impact on key economic variables but also on the rate of resource depletion and environmental deterioration

■ The hypothesis that a *conserver society* is the most basic and broad form of environmental protection

■ Corporate activities that support the principle that our environmental, energy, and economic interests converge to put a premium on greater efficiency in the industrial process

■ The need for, and nature of, a long-run integrated policy framework

■ Anticipated patterns of growth in the 1980s and the long-range trends that will inhibit growth

■ A broader perspective on the benefits of environmental regulations than on traditional economic studies

■ The ways in which environmental regulations have affected economic activity

■ The argument that environmental regulations have been the most important single force in the post-World War II era in terms of causing American industry to thoroughly rethink and often change established production processes and management practices

■ The evidence which suggests that even though the environmental regulations are not innovation oriented, they have both stimulated innovative compliance measures and have had long-term, positive effects on the general process of innovation

■ Ways in which the environmental program could explicitly foster innovation.

As a professional economist who is also deeply concerned about the long-run integrity of the environment, I am excited by the "coming together" of these two critical areas. Each has much to learn from the other—in particular, each must learn to respect the other's very legitimate demands.

The economic challenges of the 1980s are immense. Our highest priority must be to rid the economy of stagflation. We must once again

achieve reasonable levels of price stability and employment. We also must devise ways to achieve healthy economic growth rates that are sustainable over the long run. We must restore productivity vigor to the economy. We must shape an industrial structure that will ensure the United States a globally competitive export position in 1990. We must accommodate our economic-social- political system to the many ramifications of the two new transforming technologies of the 1980s: information technologies and the biotechnologies, including genetic engineering. Finally, we must learn the delicate art of balancing our economic interests with those of other nations in an increasingly interdependent, volatile global economy.

At the same time, we must move ahead vigorously on the environmental front, for the environmental problems of the 1980s are likely to prove more challenging, and in some instances more urgent, than those of ten years ago. In a sense, we have taken care of the most obvious problems: the pollutants most easy to identify and control. Now we face the more intractable environmental issues, where complexity is compounded by the fact that many are global issues requiring unprecedented forms of international cooperation. Thus, in numerous areas, both old and new, we will confront hard choices that will determine the quality of our own environment and the well-being of much of the world's population.

The first challenge is to finish the job started in the area of conventional pollutants. While we are close to 90 percent compliance with the first requirements of the Clean Air and Water Acts, the remaining sources represent around 30 to 40 percent of the environmental problem. Similarly, the wastewater treatment construction program is on the verge of major accomplishment. Congressional commitment to this program must be sustained.

The real action arenas in the 1980s will be: (1) toxics, (2) land use (including soil loss), and (3) global environmental pollution.

We have recently become aware of a whole new generation of environmental problems that are the legacy of the chemical age. Indeed, the problem of hazardous waste disposal, epitomized by the Love Canal tragedy, is the most urgent environmental challenge facing American industry today. Without swift action, we may find that in the year 2000 we have contaminated enormous amounts of our irreplaceable groundwater.

Regarding land use, positive steps must soon be taken to protect soils, safeguard critical systems and hazardous geological areas, preserve ecological and cultural diversity, and conserve the amenities of the nation's landscapes. Specifically, three of the more urgent land use problems facing the nation today are those of siting new energy facilities, protecting valuable coastal zone resources, and preserving fast-disappearing historic and cultural resources. To many observers, *3*

it now appears that in the 1980s soil erosion and the water quality problems associated with it are likely to replace petroleum as the nation's most critical natural resource problem.

One of the most vivid environmental lessons learned in the 1970s was that environmental problems do not respect national boundaries—to the contrary, many of the most serious environmental problems still remaining are inherently global in nature and will thus require global cooperation on an unprecedented scale.

The problem of running out of economically accessible, nonrenewable resources is a serious one. But it is overshadowed by the problem with renewable resource systems and the destruction of their capacity to reproduce. For example, there is increasing evidence that the global per capita productivity of each of the four natural systems (forests, fisheries, grasslands, and croplands) has peaked and is now declining. There are many specific facts that seem to indicate that this peak will not be surpassed in the foreseeable future. There are also three principal global atmospheric problems: the carbon dioxide build-up (the "greenhouse effect"), acid rain, and the depletion of the ozone layer.

The combined scope and depth of the economic and environmental challenges is immense, particularly in light of the fact that so little is known regarding the ultimate solution to any *one* problem, much less the whole confluence. What is known—or should be—is that the neglect, suspicion, and antagonism of the past between economists/business leaders and environmental scientists/environmentalists must be transformed into vigorous dialogue, acceptance, and cooperation if both the standard of living and quality of life aspirations of Americans are to be achieved. The old adage, "We must either swim together or sink together," has never been more fitting. The intent of these essays is thus to provide a first lesson in swimming together.

1

GROWTH PATTERNS AND ENVIRONMENTAL QUALITY IN THE 1980s

THE GROWTH/ ENVIRONMENT RELATIONSHIP

Throughout the 1970s, there were two opposing views regarding the alleged "growth environment trade-off." One, the most prominent in the first half of the dec-
ade, called for an end to growth, contending that growth inevitably causes a degraded environment and wasted resources. The other group, increasingly vocal in recent years, has suggested that the nation's commitment to a clean environment should be comprised in order to facilitate economic and physical growth. They argue that enforcing environmental rules will harm the economy and stall mining, construction, and manufacturing activity.

Both groups share a faulty perspective. There is no need to make either economic growth or environmental regulations a whipping boy, for the weight of evidence indicates that it is less the *fact* of growth than the *manner* of growth and the *uses* made of it which cause America's environmental troubles. For example, the introduction of a vast array of new, complex technologies, chemicals, and other materials and products in the post-World War II years—innovations that fueled the ensuing era of economic progress—was a major reason for the environmental crisis confronting the nation in 1970. The increased output of pollutants per unit of production resulting from the introduction of productive technologies since 1946 accounts for 80 to 85 percent of the total output of pollutants (except in the case of passenger travel, where it accounts for about 40 percent of the total).[1] Thus, most of the sharp increase in pollution levels has been due not so much to growth in population or affluence as to changes in productive technology. In short, the United States has largely had a counterecological pattern of growth.

Before 1970, this pattern of growth and, in particular, the value of growth were rarely questioned. Growth was discussed primarily in terms of how the growth rate could be maximized. The first overt challenge to this growth ethic came on Earth Day in April 1970. The simple message that the media carried across the United States and other industrial countries was that growth may not be all good—there may be some serious, adverse by-products (costs) that at least partially 5

offset its benefits.

Thus was born the environmental movement and the subsequent legislative and regulatory environmental initiatives. Throughout most of the 1970s, such controls were generally accepted as necessary to alleviate the high pollution levels resulting from past growth and to allow growth to continue. Still, little thought was given to the pattern of growth or to pollution prevention opportunities possible through pro-ecological growth patterns.

We must now begin such thinking as we enter the 1980s. We simply must pay more attention to *how* we are growing. Growth need not in and of itself cause pollution, nor must environmental protection necessarily limit growth. We must rid ourselves of the zero-sum mentality, for economic growth and environmental quality are not only mutually compatible but complementary in many ways. Environmental protection, for instance, goes hand-in-hand with both preserving the country's natural resource base and utilizing, in an economic fashion, existing investments in built-up as well as growing cities and metropolitan areas. Eliminating pollution will also help revitalize the nation's urban areas and reduce disparities among regions. The proper perspective is to view economic growth as a means to a quality-of-life goal, which has environmental quality as one component.

Given such an integral relationship between economic growth and environmental quality, it follows that economic development in the 1980s will be of crucial importance to the nation's environmental concerns. On the one hand, it will have direct consequences on the environment by, *inter alia,* creating new pressures and problems. It will also influence the overall social and economic climate within which environmental targets and policies will have to be formulated.

This is a particularly appropriate time to look ahead at the relationship between growth and the environment. For a number of reasons, it is likely that economic growth as traditionally measured by the GNP will be slower in the 1980s. The concurrent shift to an information economy could largely offset the inhibiting physical and social forces if managed properly. The interaction of these forces—the way we grow and the end purposes of growth—will be the crucial considerations in the managed, qualitative growth era of the 1980s and beyond.

SLOWER GROWTH AHEAD   Economic growth in the United States has always been propelled by five main engines: natural resources and the environment, human resources, capital, productivity, and technological change. From 1946 to 1966, all of these were simultaneously experiencing favorable long-run trends. In the late 1960s and early

1970s, these trends were altered. Today, they have reached the stage where each is on a new path generally not supportive of growth. For this reason, most forecasters see the 1980s as a time of slowing and generally low growth. Even the most optimistic projection, by the U.S. Department of Labor, sees a 3.6 percent average annual real growth rate for the first half of the decade declining to 3.2 percent in the second half—growth rates that are well below the more than 4 percent average for the 1960s.[2]

Slower growth is anticipated not only for the United States but for most member countries of the Organization for Economic Cooperation and Development (OECD) as well. An OECD study of medium-term developments concluded that even under favorable assumptions, growth rates of output would not return to those in the 1960s, while unemployment levels and inflation rates would remain, on average, higher than in that period.[3] The study cautioned that if economic policies are unable to fully meet the challenges before them, the industrialized world will continue to "limp along a path of relatively low growth" and unsatisfactory overall performance. The basic reason cited was that OECD economies were facing conditions that would be less supportive of growth: rising costs of raw materials; stabilizing populations; smaller productivity increases due to reduced possibilities for scale economies; a slowing of major technical innovations; and structural change, such as the increasing share of service sector employment. The report also emphasized the widespread desire among the industrialized nations for a better balance between quantitative and qualitative growth objectives.

Natural Resources and the Environment   Until the early 1970s, America was enjoying what has been characterized as a "cowboy economy," one with plenty of room to grow and few serious resource constraints. That image was shattered by two events: the birth of the environmental movement and the quadrupling of oil prices in 1973-74. Although most people expected the OPEC cartel to rapidly disintegrate, it is exerting its considerable economic muscle even more forcefully seven years later. Thus, the United States in early 1981 faces $35-$40 a barrel oil from the OPEC nations. Moreover, in recent years there has been a dramatic decline of the dollar's value in international money markets, primarily because of the huge outflow of dollars required to pay the U.S.'s oil import bill.

Two basic lessons have been learned from this experience. First, the energy crisis is primarily an oil crisis. Virtually all recent studies conclude that the production of oil will peak in the last two decades of this century. It is a virtual certainty that serious world supply-demand imbalances will appear by the 1990s. Certainly there is little optimism

regarding projected domestic oil production—most estimates show production levels in the 1990s lower than current levels. The chief dependency problem for the United States in the 1980s will be retaining access to secure sources of petroleum and natural gas. This relates closely to the second basic lesson: political realities encompassing personal ego, institutional forces, conflict, and relationships among nations have more influence on the international flow of oil than do economic factors.

Oil's dominance on the world stage may lead one to assume that there are no problems regarding other fuel and nonfuel minerals. This is not the case. Due to increased competition from other nations, the United States can no longer rely on readily available and relatively inexpensive imports as it has in the past. Indeed, a United Nations study directed by Wassily Leontief concluded that during the last 30 years of this century the world is expected to consume from three to four times as many minerals as have been consumed throughout the whole period of civilization.[4]

The question of resource availability for the United States is subject to great dispute. Although there are two polar views—one that exhaustion is inevitable and the other that humanity through its inventiveness will always be able to counteract any possible effect of scarcity—most differing opinions fall in the middle ground. The mild optimists see rising prices acting as a danger signal, discouraging the use of scarce minerals and stimulating technology and the use of alternative materials and energy sources. The mild pessimists acknowledge that the price mechanism will effectively ration scarce materials but point out that, as the fraction of the society's total resources that must be allocated to the extraction and production sector grows, there will be fewer resources available for increasing real income, since relatively fewer goods and services are produced by the lowered resource base.

As the United States is forced to move to continually lower grade resources, a self-accelerating power/resource demand cycle emerges. In the energy sector, increasing dependence on lower-grade energy sources for the extraction of power will, of itself, demand increasing power and increasing amounts of manufactured goods. In the manufacturing sector, the demand for more manufactured goods just to convert available energy to usable power consumes more raw resources and increases power consumption in the manufacturing process. In the raw materials sector, the increasing demand by manufacturing processes for refined raw materials from lower and lower grade sources will, of itself, cause an increase in the power and manufactured goods demanded for raw resource extraction and refinement. In short, the action of every sector increases the rate of

reaction of all sectors so that even if consumer demands remain

constant, the rate of resource consumption accelerates. Stated somewhat differently, the rate at which our resource reserves diminish will continue to increase even if human populations stabilize and average per capita consumptions levels off.

Thus, the United States is confronted with a serious race between technological progress and the economic depletion of its resource endowment—and even resource availability through imports—due to burgeoning worldwide demand. To date, technology has been the victor, and many argue that the new technologies which will arise and help increase efficiency in extracting and using resources will also be sufficient. Most observers, however, would agree that it is far from clear that these technologies will be able to offset the hard fact that, due to continuing resource depletion, given inputs of labor, capital, energy, and other factor inputs will yield less output of energy and resources. Certainly, unproductive U.S. efforts to develop commercially available synthetic fuels or oil shale should prompt us to be cautious.

What does seem likely to occur during the last two decades of this century is a substantial increase in the real cost of most natural resources due to both "imperfections" in market systems and institutional arrangements. In addition, many of the real costs involved in present mineral production and consumption will be paid in the future, and the United States' fuel and nonfuel mineral import dependency, which is already high, will likely be substantially higher in the year 2000.

Though resource scarcity and resource exhaustion were much discussed throughout the 1970s, the major natural resource problem of today is how to strike a balance between growth and protection of the environment. It is a problem well known to the public through constant press exposure: the siting of electrical plants, the laying of pipelines in Alaska, the disposal of nuclear wastes, the problem of automobile emissions, the pollution of lakes and rivers, urban noise levels, and so on.

It thus has the potential to constrain both the rate and pattern of economic growth. These constraints come primarily in the form of limits to the absorptive capacity of the environment and the costs borne by industries and other institutions to limit their pollution emittants. First, however, let's take a look at the services provided by the environment.

Foremost among these services is a generally hospitable habitat for humans and other forms of life. The environment is the source of all material inputs to the economy, including fuels and minerals, air and water. It also provides amenities, such as places where one goes for vacations, weekend outings, or walks. Finally, its services include residuals absorption or waste reception. These are all economic goods in that, other things being equal, people are willing to pay to receive

more or to avoid a reduction in quality or the quantity of the service.

Economic analysis has been particularly faulty in regard to the absorptive capacity of the environment. Most economic analysis of environmental pollution has implicitly assumed a constant available absorptive capacity of common property resources to assimilate the residuals from consumption and production activities. This assumption runs contrary to scientific evidence. Some economic activities result in the depletion of the stock (or capacity) of common property resources that yield various life support services. The burning of fossil fuels, for example, by producing carbon dioxides and releasing fine particulates that absorb heat, holds real prospects of altering the mean global temperature—with potentially catastrophic results. The use of fluorocarbons in refrigeration, and also the release of oxides of nitrogen from the practice of intensive agriculture, deplete the capacity of the ozone layer to filter out carcinogenic solar radiations. By altering the composition of the atmosphere, economic activity depletes common property resources, which are vital constituents of our life support system.

It is also clear that past treatment of the environment has given the wrong signals for the directions of economic growth. These wrong signals stem from the simple fact that the market principle has never been applied to the use of air and water. By treating many things as free that were not really free, we were in effect subsidizing various goods, resulting in their overproduction. Factoring in the environment, either through standards or various economic incentives, such as the offset market, will change future patterns of growth.

Human Resources

One of the most dramatic changes among the traditional sources of growth in the 1980s will be the sharp slowdown in labor force growth and a basic shift in its age distribution. Due to the sharp drop in the birth rate during the late 1950s and early 1960s, the increase in the size of the labor force in the 1980s will be less than 12 percent (compared to a growth of nearly 21 percent in the 1970s). The drop in the birth rate means that the percentage of 18-24 year olds in the working age population group (18-64 year old population) will decline from 22.1 percent in 1975 to 16.9 percent in 1990. This translates into a decline in the growth rate of the working-age population from an annual rate of 1.8 percent during the 1970s to only 1.0 percent during the 1980s— about as slow a rate of growth for a ten-year period as ever experienced in the United States. The Bureau of Labor Statistics projects that the rate of labor force growth will average 2.1 percent per year during 1977-80, 1.6 percent during 1980-85, and 1.1 percent during 1985-90.[5]

This slowing in the growth of the labor force will have two major effects, both conducive to productivity. Since the incidence of

unemployment tends to decline with age, an older, more experienced work force is expected to be both more productive and less prone to joblessness. Slower labor force growth should also raise the cost of labor relative to capital, causing a shift toward labor-raising capital investment. This would reverse the sharp deterioration in the nation's capital-labor ratio, and should help boost productivity.

Capital, Productivity, and Technological Change   These three factors, being so closely inter-related, should be considered together. Each of them had a dismal performance record in the 1970s compared to the two previous decades. The serious decline in the labor productivity growth rate is well known. For the decade as a whole, it averaged 1.3 percent annually, less than one half the 3.0 percent annual rate of increase during the 1960s. Not as well known is the equally serious decline in the productivity of capital. From 1947-66, the output/capital ratio increased at an average rate of 0.5 percent per year, while from 1967-74 it actually fell an average 1.3 percent per year. This decline may continue because of the increasing rate of equipment obsolescence. The falling ratio is a key contributor to the general expectation that capital expenditures in the 1980s will likely be insufficient to generate enough capacity to meet the demands of the economy—including national goals in the areas of employment, productivity, domestic energy production, pollution abatement, and healthful working conditions—at reasonably stable prices. The result will be bottlenecks and sporadic shortages.

It has become fashionable to speak woefully of the decline of technology in America. Proponents of this technology decline argument have been able to marshal an impressive array of supporting evidence and statistics. These are highlighted in the opening section of Chapter 4, "Environmental Regulation and Technological Innovation."

THE NEW INFORMATION ECONOMY

The Dynamic Elements of the Transformation   The microprocessor (or computer-on-a-chip) best symbolizes the dynamic structural transformation of the U.S. economy currently taking place. It has been called the engine that is powering a second industrial revolution, and the single invention that is most radically altering U.S. industry. It is said to be rewriting the economics of computing and will eventually become as basic to industry as steel is. It can increase typing efficiency fourfold or more and has made possible the creation of electronic robots that can "see" moving parts on a conveyor belt, pick them up, and transfer them to another location.

This is an example par excellence of a "radical breakthrough" in   *11*

technological innovation, which has been so conspicuously absent in the past 10-15 years. Microprocessors cannot be treated as just another family of components but must be seen as full-blown computer systems, requiring new approaches to product definition and design, new engineering and marketing skills, new business strategies, and, in many cases, separate organizations.

That the information revolution is very much with us can be seen in the following statistics: by 1955, information workers had surpassed industrial workers as the dominant category in the labor force; by 1967, the total information activity—meaning the resources consumed in producing, processing, and distributing information goods and services—accounted for 46 percent of the GNP; currently, more than half of the workers in the United States are primarily engaged in generating, processing, distributing, analyzing, or otherwise handling information.[6]

The future promises continued rapid growth in the computer-electronics-telecommunication arena due to an anticipated outpouring of new technological innovations and applications. Through 1985, the installed population of computers and terminals is projected to grow at a compound annual rate of more than 30 percent. Because the price/performance ratio in electronics decreases dramatically, the information processing capability of the U.S. economy can be expected to increase by a compound annual rate greater than 100 percent.

Nor is such dynamic activity confined solely to the United States. Indeed, electronics has been one of the most rapidly expanding sectors throughout the world during the last decade, with a growth rate of physical output of more than 10 percent per annum between 1965 and 1975. It is, therefore, not surprising that a 1979 OECD report on the long-run future of its member countries concluded:

> Through its links with data processing and telecommunications, the introduction of automation throughout industry, the changes which electronic office equipment is producing in service activities, and the actual services which it creates, the electronics complex will during the next quarter of a century be the main pole around which the productive structures of the advanced industrial societies will be reorganized.[7]

In sharp contrast to this dynamic, innovative activity, most of the basic, or heavy, industries have "matured" and thus are experiencing a relative decline in importance, which will continue into the 1980s. A major study of 2,500 corporations in 37 industries found less and less new investment money going into such industries, especially manufacturing industries and in particular the basic industries that largely produce capital goods.[8] The best case in point is steel, where

investment had fallen to a 6 percent annual rate of growth in the period 1966-76, compared to more than 10 percent for industry as a whole.

Although these industries are experiencing a *relative* decline, they will still be very much with us. Thus, the transformation from an industrial-based economy to an "information economy" does not mean that the society is less technologically based or is moving beyond industry, but simply that the production/manufacturing industries become less important as the prime motive force and wealth-generating sector. The characteristics of the central technologies and industrial forms become inherently different.

The Implications of the Transformation   The "information revolution," as it is increasingly called, could ultimately lead to socioeconomic change more far reaching than that wrought by the Industrial Revolution. The two revolutions are quite different, and their fundamental difference is of profound significance for environmental quality in the 1980s.

Whereas the Industrial Revolution made available and employed vast amounts of mechanical energy, the information revolution is extremely sparing of energy and materials. Much of industrial technology was crude, with only a modest scientific or theoretical base. The information revolution, as the product of the most advanced science, technology, and management, represents one of the greatest intellectual achievements of mankind.

The Industrial Revolution, highly dependent on large quantities of increasingly scarce energy and raw materials, will be limited by the paucity or high price of these necessary ingredients. The information revolution, fueled by silicon (one of the most abundant elements on earth) and by intellectual achievements, is destined for long-continued growth as its knowledge base inevitably increases.

The impact of the shift to an information economy will be pervasive, affecting how and what we produce, how we transact business, how we communicate and pay our bills, where we work, and even what kind of work we do. Not restricted to just the computer or communications industries, the information revolution embraces banking, insurance, transportation, health, education, communications, entertaining, and manufacturing. Given such a wide range of impacts in so many different industries, all the key economic variables will clearly be affected. But the greatest and most direct impacts will be on productivity, employment, and trade.

CHANGING VALUES   In early 1979, Daniel Yankelovich and Bernard Lefkowitz examined a wide body of social research data showing the attitudes, beliefs, and values of Americans regarding the prospects for economic growth and its   *13*

consequences. Their research revealed a picture of Americans "midway between an older post-World War II attitude of expanding horizons, a growing psychology of entitlement, unfettered optimism, and unqualified confidence in technology and economic growth, and a present state of mind of lowering expectations, apprehensions about the future, mistrust in institutions, and a growing psychology of limits."[9]

Thus, the transformation that America is currently undergoing does not consist solely of change in the underlying economic structure; equally important is a substantial change in the values, attitudes, and priorities of the American people.

Increasing Skepticism Concerning Growth As evident from the above quote, Americans are very confused in their thinking about growth. They are weighing the arguments, pro and con, and assessing the virtues and drawbacks of economic expansion. They are uncertain what concessions or sacrifices they will have to make if they enlist on one side or the other.

Recent surveys and changes in lifestyle have made it clear, however, that in contrast to the first 25 years after World War II, the American people are increasingly skeptical about the nation's capacity for unlimited economic growth, are becoming wary of the benefits unlimited economic growth is supposed to bring, and are beginning to place a higher priority on improving human and social relationships than on raising the material standard of living. What has caused such a turnabout in values?

At the most basic level, growth does not adequately address the fundamental requirements common to all humans:

- Basic human needs ("enough" food, shelter, health, education, employment, and security)
- A sense of the dignity of being human
- A sense of becoming (a chance to achieve a better life)
- A sense of justice or equity
- A sense of achievement, related to something worth achieving
- A sense of solidarity, of belonging to a worthy group, and of participation in decisions that affect the group's, and one's own, destiny

In short, growth has not brought the promised contentment or fulfillment. Most Americans have acquired an abundance of material things, yet remain vexed, not only by the immediate economic and noneconomic problems in their individual personal lives, but by larger
issues that extend outward to embrace the whole society and forward

to encompass the future. An increasing number now view quality of life not simply as a vision of an overflowing cornucopia of personal material luxuries, but as something less tangible and yet more important—job satisfaction, a healthy environment, good schools, responsive and efficient government, and fulfilling leisure activities.

The value change has also resulted from the public's growing awareness that scientific and technological advance is a double-edged sword that threatens man and his environment while at the same time offering the tempting vision of a better future. As knowledge of the delicate interwebbing of the ecological system has spread, people have demanded wide-ranging measures to protect the natural environment. As the carcinogenic nature of some industrial products and processes has been recognized, the demand for other protective measures has risen. Current apprehension about the ultimate physical and social consequences of nuclear power technology may retard a development that until recently was expected to yield a cornucopia of benefits. Research into genetic manipulations also has aroused new reservations about the independence of science.

Demands for Environmental Protection   It can be soundly argued that the change in values has been most clearly manifested in the environmental movement of the 1970s. Before the 1970s, certain fundamental premises stemming from the prevailing values of the industrial era contributed to the massive environmental problems faced in 1970 and still faced today:

■   That humans are essentially distinct from nature, and hence that nature is to be exploited and "controlled" rather than cooperated with
■   That humans are basically "economic animals," and that therefore economic policy should give priority to an ever-increasing GNP, material consumption, and expenditure of irreplaceable resources
■   That humans are essentially separate from one another, so that little intrinsic responsibility is felt for the effects of present actions on remote individuals or future generations

Certainly, these views have contributed to greater and greater disruption of previous ecological balances, ravaging of the environment, and squandering of natural resources.

The widespread challenge to these premises began in the late 1960s and culminated on Earth Day in April 1970. It is clear that the Environmental Protection Agency, which began operation in December 1970, did not come into being simply because a few administration officials or members of Congress thought the country needed it. Rather, it was the direct result of changed values and   *15*

priorities.

In the midst of high inflation and general economic difficulties, one might expect the public to be abandoning strong environmental values. Yet this has not occurred. A comprehensive National Environmental Survey conducted in late 1978 found that more than half the people think protecting the environment is so important that "continuing improvements must be made regardless of cost."[10] Contrary to the white, upper-middle-class image of environmental concern, black support (55 percent) was virtually identical to that of whites (54 percent), and 49 percent of those with very low incomes (under $6,000) chose this option. By three to one, the respondents favored paying higher prices to protect the environment over paying lower prices but putting up with more air and water pollution.

The finding that Americans strongly favor environmental protection despite its large costs is not unique to this poll. According to Lou Harris, the results of his polling on environmental-energy trade-offs can be summarized by this message from the public to policymakers: "Don't you dare relax your all-out efforts to make certain that environmental hazards are kept to an absolute minimum." The Opinion Research Corporation wrote in its Report to Management (February 1977), "It would be foolish for anyone to conclude that the public is less than adamant about environmental quality."

The Gap Between *Attitudes and Behavior* A number of studies have documented a change in people's values regarding material progress and their consumption levels. Studies conducted between 1968-78 by the University of Michigan's Survey Research Center show that, for the average family, the following priorities gained in importance at the expense of an increase in the level of consumption: a secure job; continuous income even in case of sickness, disability, and old age; appropriate forms of job and career; safety in one's home and on the street; and neighborhoods that do not deteriorate as the result of rapid changes in the human or physical environment.[11]

Attitudes, however, do not necessarily translate into behavior. Indeed, over the past seven years, while awareness of shortages and of limits has grown, conserving behavior has actually decreased. Consider what has happened in the arena that offers the ultimate challenge to American willpower—the auto. Roper found in 1974 that 52 percent of respondents reported using their cars less often than in the past; this number diminished to 33 percent in 1976. Similarly, Yankelovich. Skelly and White (YSW) found that the 61 percent majority that reported taking fewer nonessential car trips in 1974 than *16* in earlier years had been slashed to a 36 percent minority in 1978.

Concerning driving at lower speeds, Roper found 71 percent reported doing so in 1974 but only 56 percent in 1976, while YSW found that their 1974 figure of 72 percent had shrunk to 60 percent in 1978. In the 1974-79 period, YSW also showed a net decline in the number of people reporting that they: keep a car longer before getting a new one (69 percent to 61 percent); keep thermostats at lower temperatures than in earlier years (67 percent to 63 percent); are more careful with clothing, which they keep longer or patch up before discarding (60 percent to 48 percent); and save things, such as empty jars, containers and wrappings, that they would normally throw away (55 percent to 43 percent).

Such results led Yankelovich and Lefkowitz to conclude: "Americans speak enthusiastically about the moral benefits of the simple non-materialistic life. But they have yet to fully incorporate these benefits either in their day-to-day behavior or in their practical thinking and planning for the future."[12]

This finding is undoubtedly true for the vast majority of Americans. However, there are an estimated 4 to 5 million adults who are already practicing a lifestyle that has been called "voluntary simplicity"—an effort to live life within a new balance between inner and outer growth.[13] It embraces frugality of consumption, a strong sense of environmental urgency, a desire to return to living and working environments that are on a more human scale, and an intention to realize our higher human potential in community with others. It means living simply not just because prices are rising, but because you value conservation in and of itself. The five values that seem to lie at the heart of this emerging way of life are material simplicity, human scale, self-determination, ecological awareness, and personal growth.

Toward a Resolution   The American psyche is in a very critical period. Traditional values, attitudes, and priorities are crumbling with no clear replacements in sight. It is little wonder that in 1978, for the first time, Americans believed that the past was a better time than the present, and they anticipated that the present, however bad, is likely to be better than the future. This is a historic shift from traditional American optimism to an uncharacteristically bleak outlook.

George Katona has pinpointed the primary reason for this shift: "What demarcates the 1970s from the fifties and sixties is that in the current era, public confidence in the government—and especially in the effectiveness of government economic policy—has practically vanished, and as it has, economic confidence has also crumbled."[14] The decline of confidence, according to Yankelovich and Lefkowitz, has been "swift, sharp, and all-encompassing."

In 1964 a 69% majority of the American public had faith in the competence of government officials ("They know what they are doing"); by 1976 the number of Americans holding this view dropped to 44%; by 1978 it had dropped further to 40%.

At the end of the 1950s, a 56% majority of the public expressed the view that "you can trust the government in Washington to do what is right most of the time." Two decades later their level of trust had been cut virtually in half to 29%.

In the mid 1960s, by a more than two to one margin (64% to 28%) Americans believed that the government was run for all the people rather than for the benefit of a few big interests. By 1978, this pattern had completely reversed itself by an almost three to one margin (65% to 23%).

The number of Americans believing that the Federal Government is "getting too powerful for the good of the country" has increased over approximately a quarter of a century from a 42% minority to a 68% majority.[15]

The public has been shown to be pessimistic, disillusioned, and highly uncertain about the future. Yet, opinion survey data also suggest that at a deeper level of consciousness Americans have begun to reconcile themselves to the need to accept greater, and different, limits than in the past. The stage is thus set for the nation to move toward some resolution of what it has to give up and what it insists upon retaining.

Yankelovich and Lefkowitz propose three overall conditions for forming a resolution. The first, and perhaps most important, is that the country has to feel the necessity for making hard choices. These choices cannot be abstract or theoretical, and people must believe that their decisions will have a direct, immediate, and significant effect on their lives. A second vital precondition is political leadership that will define the terms of the debate and propose real choices and national priorities for the future. The final one is that the public be given the opportunity to confront and think through the real choices. Resolution will only be possible if average Americans feel they are part of the decision-making continuum, if they feel that their point of view is heard and responded to, and if they feel that their fundamental values are respected.

FOOTNOTES TO CHAPTER 1

1. Barry Commoner, *The Closing Circle,* New York: Alfred A. Knopf, 1972, p. 176.

2. Valerie A. Personick, "Industry Output and Employment: BLS Projections to 1980," *Monthly Labor Review,* April 1979, p. 4.

3. Organization for Economic Cooperation and Development; *Facing the Future,* Paris, 1979.

4. Wassily Leontief, *The Future of the World Economy,* New York: United Nations, 1977, p. 22.

5. Personick, op. cit., p. 4.

6. These statistics are drawn from the seminal work on this topic by Marc Porat, *The Information Economy: Definition and Measurement,* U.S. Department of Commerce, Office of Telecommunication, O.T. Special Publication 77-12(1), May 1977.

7. OECD, op. cit., p. 336.

8. The survey was done for Business Week by Investors Management Sciences, Inc. and was highlighted in "The Slow Investment Economy," *Business Week,* October 17, 1977.

9. Daniel Yankelovich and Bernard Lefkowitz, "The Public Debate on Growth: Preparing for Resolution," paper for Third Biennial Woodlands Conference on Growth Policy, Houston, October 1979.

10. Robert Cameron Mitchell, "The Public Speaks Again: A New Environmental Survey," *Resources,* September-November 1978.

11. George Katona and Burkhard Strumpel, *A New Economic Era,* New York: Elsevier, 1978.

12. Yankelovich and Lefkowitz, op. cit., p. 38.

13. Duane S. Elgin and Arnold Mitchell, "Voluntary Simplicity: Lifestyle of the Future?", *Futurist,* August 1977.

14. Cited in Yankelovich and Lefkowitz, op. cit., p. 19.

15. Yankelovich and Lefkowitz, op. cit., pp. 34-5.

2

A CONSERVER SOCIETY TO ENHANCE ENVIRONMENTAL QUALITY

QUALITATIVE GROWTH AS THE GOAL President Carter's unprecedented address to the nation in July 1979 spoke of a "crisis of confidence" in which Americans' trust in virtually all institutions and particularly government had plummeted throughout the 1970s. Americans no longer believed the future would be better for them and their children—a dramatic reversal of the historically prevailing national spirit.

Given such a fundamental malaise, Carter's prescription was remarkably narrow in focus. It appeared as though energy held the key to everything, that if tens of billions of dollars were spent in the 1980s to reduce U.S. dependence on foreign oil, the malaise would be lifted by 1990.

Such a vigorous effort to boost domestic energy production and cut energy demand is vitally needed. Though necessary, however, it is far from sufficient to relieve the larger crisis of confidence, which has much deeper roots. A large part of the problem may be that the economic problem—defined by Keynes as the struggle for subsistence—has been solved in the United States. If one accepts, as Keynes did, that "we have been expressly evolved by nature—with all our impulses and deepest instincts—for the purpose of solving the economic problem," then we as a nation have been deprived of our previous central purpose.

Moreover, we have become a fractionated society characterized by the absence of a shared system of values. As was said of ancient Rome, we "tolerate few or no restraints on the feverish struggle of contending appetites... There [is] no longer any body of sound opinion to which, in the last resort, appeal [can] be made."

It is little wonder that an exhaustive survey of recent public opinion polls revealed a picture of Americans "midway between an older post-World War II attitude of expanding horizons, a growing psychology of entitlement, unfettered optimism, and unqualified confidence in technology and economic growth, and a present state of mind of lowering expectations, apprehensions about the future, mistrust in institutions, and a growing psychology of limits."[1]

It is clear that Americans have become quite confused in their attitude regarding growth and material progress. They are increasingly skeptical about the nation's capacity for unlimited economic growth, are becoming wary of the benefits unlimited economic growth is supposed to bring, and are beginning to place a higher priority on improving human and social relationships than on raising the material standard of living.

A primary reason for this turnabout in values is that growth has not brought contentment or fulfillment to life. The vast majority of Americans have acquired an abundance of material things yet remain vexed, not only by the immediate noneconomic problems in their individual personal lives but by larger issues that extend outward to embrace the whole society and forward to encompass the future. An increasing number now view quality of life not simply as a vision of an overflowing cornucopia of personal material luxuries, but as something less tangible and yet more important—job satisfaction, good schools, responsive government, fulfilling leisure activities. The American public needs a positive vision of America in the 1980s— where we are headed as a nation and why, and what the concrete steps (or alternatives) are to get us there. People's serious questioning of the value of growth and their growing expression of diverse quality-of-life concerns indicates the type of vision that should be put forth by political leaders as a major challenge for America to meet in the 1980s: a vision of qualitative, selective growth to replace the present allegiance to quantitative, undifferentiated growth. A three-to-one majority in a Harris poll endorsed the statement, "The trouble with most leaders is that they don't understand people want better quality of almost everything they have rather than more quantity."

The new questions must ask about purposes: Growth for whom? Growth for what? An expanded GNP goal must not be automatically applauded before we ask: How will the growth be achieved and what ends will it serve? Growth must come to be seen as a means to an end and not the end itself.

At a minimum, we must move in the 1980s toward an economic growth that is restrained by sound environmental-physical principles and that is both sustainable and productive of desirable human ends. Redirecting future economic growth into nonpolluting and resource-conserving channels will help minimize its disruptive effects upon the environment. The broader objective of policy must be to maximize national economic welfare, defined to take account of pollution, resource depletion, the quality of work, income distribution, and other aspects of welfare not reflected in the GNP as now calculated.

The strategic question is: What does it mean in practical terms to pursue a qualitative growth goal? What specific actions and policies will be involved?

The wide array of actions and policies that would be involved in pursuing qualitative growth can be grouped under two main guiding principles, which relate to physical resources and human resources. In the physical realm, the actions and policies of corporations and governments should conform to a "conserver society" goal, one that requires the use of the minimum amount of resources deemed necessary to carry out an activity or produce a product (including growth) without resulting in undesirable side effects. The guiding principle for human resources should be total employment, wherein everyone desiring a job would have the opportunity of obtaining one that essentially satisfies his or her personal desires.

In addition to conserving resources and energy, a conserver society should contribute greatly to the achievement of enhanced environmental quality in the 1980s. Indeed, the resulting, redirected patterns of growth constitute the most basic and wide-ranging form of environmental protection, for it has not been growth per se, but the manner of growth and the uses made of it, that are the root of U.S. environmental troubles. Indeed, a major reason for the environmental crisis that the United States faced in 1970 was that the progress of the 1950s and 1960s was achieved through the introduction of a vast array of often environmentally destructive complex technologies, chemicals, and other materials and products. Since the sharp increase in pollution levels has been due not so much to population increase or affluence as to changes in productive technology, it can be concluded that the United States has largely had a counterecological pattern of growth. A conserver society would employ a wide variety of measures to help reverse this pattern.

This improvement in environmental quality would not come at the expense of growth. In fact, in helping to assure adequate supplies of energy and mineral resources, a conserver society is the only basis for sustained economic growth over the long-run. Conserver principles reconcile the environment with the economy—our ends with our means.

A CONSERVER SOCIETY AS THE MEANS

Basic Principles

The basic idea behind the conserver society is the notion of conservation, which can be defined as the process of prolonging (either by preserving or by using-and-recycling) the useful life of resources. Basic questions to address are: (1) What do we wish to conserve? (2) For how long a period? (3) Who are the beneficiaries of this conservation and who are the losers, if any?

The United States has flirted with certain features of a conserver society in the past. A conserver-society concept, for instance, is found in the writings of Emerson and Thoreau and in the work of the Hudson

Valley painters. At times, it even found expression in political life; for example, just before the turn of century when Congress established Yosemite as the world's first national park, or when President Theodore Roosevelt, on his last night in office, preempted for national conservation half of what is now the national park system.

But by and large, the United States has not been a conserving nation; the growth and resource-exploitation ethic has dominated decisions by business and government. In addition, the government has never had a comprehensive natural resources policy that seeks to use judiciously our declining supply of domestic natural resources and available imports.

Most people today would readily identify conservation with energy conservation. The conserver society, however, would encompass the conservation of all natural resources and raw materials. The basic idea would be to effect transition from a "linear" economy, in which extracted resources move through production processes and are ultimately disposed of as waste in some form, to a "circular" one in which a substantial proportion of output would be recycled for further production, instead of discarded as rubbish. Instead of maximizing the throughput in the system and supporting the value of built-in obsolescence, the economy would produce long-lasting quality goods to meet genuine human needs. As expressed by E. F. Schumacher, "From an economic point of view, the central concept of wisdom is permanence. We must study the economics of permanence."[2]

In addition to simply increasing the lifetime of products and reducing demand for material-intensive products or services, there are a number of other means of conservation: cutting waste generation in production; reducing the amount of material embodied in the product; recycling; and materials substitution. The potential of each of these means depends upon developments in technology, economic incentives, changes in lifestyle, and changes in product specification. The goal should be to attain an efficient balance among them.

Talbot Page has succinctly phrased the key questions:

> By what standards do we judge the best, or optimal, balance between depletion and conservation of materials, between disposal and recycling, durability and original cost, maintenance and new production? These questions lead directly to another: How should we account for the very long-run costs which may be associated with materials depletion and waste generation.[3]

Feasibility

Before proceeding, the critical question of whether a conserver society is feasible must be addressed. The specific and most common form this question has taken is, will significant cutbacks in energy use resulting from

energy conservation measures curtail or even cripple economic growth? Indeed, the fear of such a relationship has been a principal reason why the United States has not launched a serious energy conservation program in the six years since the OPEC oil embargo. That the lower energy-lower growth argument is heard so often is surprising in light of so much evidence to the contrary.

Researchers at Resources for the Future, on the basis of an in-depth quantitative study, concluded that the argument is false on historical grounds—there has been no such inviolable relationship between energy and GNP growth.[4] In addition, the experience of other industrialized countries provides current evidence that no such relationship exists. A major study on comparative energy use in industrialized countries found that the North American countries consume on an average about 50 percent more energy relative to GNP than the countries of Western Europe and Japan.[5] The higher U.S. energy consumption is reflected in almost all sectors. Finally, virtually all recent studies examining the future of the energy-GNP relationship have concluded that energy growth could be substantially cut without seriously affecting economic growth prospects. A Conference Board study found annual GNP growth of 3.5 percent consistent with annual 1.5 percent energy growth, while the Institute for Energy Analysis put GNP growth with this energy level at 1.5 to 3.0 percent; Dale Jorgenson concluded that each percentage point reduction in energy input leads only to a 0.2 percentage point reduction in real GNP; and William Nordhaus found that if energy demand in the year 2010 were 73 quads, actually less than the 78 quads in 1978, this would reduce real income by only 2.3 percent.[6]

Energy conservation is not only feasible but also economically smart, as it is generally cheaper than investment in new energy supplies. The international experts at the 1976 Bellagio Conference on Science, Technology, and Society concluded that in a rising cost environment, "conservation will make more economic sense than an increase in supplies in many more instances than has been true in the past."[7] Certainly it is true that, to the degree that clean air and water and land itself have become increasingly scarce and costly goods, it makes both environmental and economic sense to make the conservation of energy and the reduction or recovery of waste a matter of the highest priority.

Indeed, a vigorous energy conservation program would simultaneously optimize economic, energy, and environmental policy goals. It would, for example, slow down the required rate of capital formation for high-technology energy development and, therefore, would exert an anti-inflationary impact. This slowdown would also allow for greater flexibility and balance in the allocation of capital to social, economic, and environmental goals. In addition, conservation

methods and renewable energy sources are labor-intensive rather than energy- and capital-intensive and thus are excellent generators of jobs. The American Institute of Architects projects that between 500,000 and 1 million new jobs would result from a conservation program for new and old buildings through 1990. Labor intensiveness and decentralization provide the ancillary advantage of greater opportunities for small business, indigenous business, and community enterprises. In general, the combined policy of conservation and renewables buys time, allowing the energy R&D program to devise solutions that will overcome the technical barriers to the more complete utilization of renewable energy technologies such as solar power generation.

Because energy has become such an urgent matter, it is likely that energy conservation will eventually become an ingrained habit of American life. But what are the chances of the United States ever becoming a conserver society on a broader scale? Could a nation even seriously consider moving in that direction?

In the mid-1970s, the Science Council of Canada explored the concept of a conserver society in a series of reports. Its first report in 1973 recommended that "Canadians as individuals, and their governments, institutions and industries begin the transition from a consumer society preoccupied with resource exploitation to a conserver society engaged in more constructive endeavors."[8] The general dimensions of such a society were outlined by a Science Council Committee in 1975 that was established to direct a study on "The Implications of a Conserver Society."

A conserver society is in principle against waste and pollution. Therefore, it is a society that:

■ Promotes economy of design of all systems, i.e., "doing more with less"
■ Favors reuse of recycling and, wherever possible, reduction at source
■ Questions the ever-growing per capita demand for consumer goods, artificially encouraged by modern marketing techniques, and
■ Recognizes that a diversity of solutions in many systems, such as energy and transportation, might in effect increase their overall economy, stability, and resiliency.[9]

A 1976 report showed Canada in the longer run becoming a conserver society using food, energy, and resources frugally and using transportation and communications technology to permit a very wide choice of lifestyle, often in small communities.

The United States as a Prototype   The United States, consuming as it does such a large (one may say disproportionate) share of the world's resources, could exercise considerable global leadership through pursuit of a conserver society goal. If the United States established an ecologically sound, resource-conserving growth pattern, it would have an impact on the availability of resources to the rest of the world in proportion to the huge share of those resources which the country now consumes. It also could serve as a prototype of new societal development for other advanced industrialized nations struggling with the adverse by-products of economic growth and dwindling or increasingly expensive natural resources. Thus, as the United States moved toward becoming a conserver society, its international position would be improved both in terms of its image and its increasingly interdependent future.

Whether the United States can become a conserver society depends primarily on the values, attitudes, and priorities adopted by the people. Since most problems that beset our society encroach gradually and are caused by the day-to-day behavior of individuals, they can ultimately be resolved only by a change in that behavior. It has been argued that during the next two decades American will be *forced* to learn to live with new scarcities and to acquire habits of personal and social thrift. Yankelovich and Lefkowitz, however, found from their survey of public opinion polls taken over the past five years that the American public may be at the leading edge of the conservation ethic. Although people are not ready to give up those things they consider essential to their well-being and freedom (their cars, central heating, washing machines), they are prepared to make modest cutbacks in the use of energy, to keep their cars longer, to reduce consumption of meat and clothing, and to reduce their use of items that cannot be recycled if these involve waste. Based on such data, Yankelovich and Lefkowitz see a movement toward a more conserving society that is being accelerated by three significant psychosocial developments: the heightened emphasis on economic security, lowered economic expectations, and new values. They, therefore, conclude that one of the four major "ideological forms" of the future will be "a more conserving society with a greater balance than now exists between consumption and nonmaterialistic values."[10]

The United States has before it the option to create a society that has conserver values, that runs on renewable energy, that recycles many of its materials, that is wholly sustainable and regenerative. Within a decade perhaps, surely by the year 2000, we could be viewed as a conserver society. This does not imply some static state, for the conserver society is really a process, a conceptual force that opens up options in order to keep them open, not to fix our destiny to one
particular narrow vision. Being flexible, a conserver society can be

achieved through many means; once in place, it can be made to respond to many needs. It prescribes nothing but a framework within which infinite combinations of conserving actions can interact. The current and potential actions and policies of corporations and government, described in the remainder of this chapter, provide one set of available options.

THE ROLE OF CORPORATIONS AND MARKET FORCES

Milton Friedman has succinctly expressed the traditional perspective on corporations' social responsibility: "There is one and only one social responsibility of business—to use its resources and engage in activities to increase its profits."[11] An opposing viewpoint, developed in the 1970s, argues that corporations, as creatures of the state, have an explicit responsibility to conform to broad societal goals. This view has been expounded not only by those outside the business community and critical of its ways but by an increasing number of corporate leaders. Louis Lundborg, former chairman of the board of the Bank of America, argues strongly that corporate leadership should be responsive to environmental and social concerns: "Those in corporate life are going to be expected to do things for the good of society just to earn their franchise, their corporate right to exist."[12] He believes that debating the issues of corporate social responsibility is nonsense: "Environmental and other social problems should get at least as much corporate attention as production, sales, and finance. The quality of life in its total meaning is, in the final reckoning, the only justification for any corporate activity."[13]

The likely counterresponse would be: "That is all well and good in theory; but in practice, production, sales, and finance would suffer." The notion that pollution control or resource conservation practices have to be a burden to the firm, ultimately lowering profits, is widespread but false.

Basically, what companies have been discovering in recent years is that waste is just that—waste—and if it can be eliminated or, better yet, creatively utilized, it will benefit the bottom line. Indeed, it is creative use of waste—the most obvious being recycling and energy conservation—that lies at the heart of most conserver society practices.

Corporate Activities to Date

A considerable amount of recycling is being done at the present time. It is ironic that "junk" materials for recycling supplied the nation in the mid 1970s with 44 percent of its copper, 20 percent of its iron and steel, almost 50 percent of its lead, and about 20 percent of its paper. The U.S. recovery rate for copper is the best in the world, and the high rate for lead is especially remarkable since several

hundred thousand tons of lead are devoted annually to dissipative uses, the largest being gasoline additives.

Certainly significant energy conservation efforts are also underway. Industry officials in 1978 reported that energy conservation was about the most profitable use for their capital, causing companies to spend hundreds of millions of dollars. For instance:

> Scientists at a half dozen other respected companies, including General Electric, are also sketching windmills these days. Elsewhere in the white-smocked reaches of the nation's corporate laboratories, researchers are trying to squeeze power from ocean heat, design hollow ball bearings to cut auto weight, and convert wood chips from logged-over forests into fuel oil. Such projects, implausible or even ludicrous just five years ago, are evidence of the most far-reaching transformation to hit company research labs in more than a decade. Energy worries are sparking a basic reorientation of corporate research and development.[14]

Furthermore, rapidly rising spending in this area, currently adding to total capital outlays, will be increasingly important in the next few years. Dow Chemical, for instance, has projected over $200 million of energy-saving investment opportunities in its Texas and Louisiana facilities alone, each project offering a greater than 50 percent pretax return on investment.

Corporations have also been eliminating or utilizing wastes in ways not well known to the public. In the past few years, an increasing number of U.S. firms have undertaken process changes in response to environmental regulations, which have resulted in net economic and/or energy savings. A prime example is the 3M Company's Pollution Prevention Pays program. Corporate officials introduced it in 1975 to stress conservation-oriented technology that will prevent pollution at the source in products and manufacturing processes rather than remove pollution after it is created. To date, 39 projects selected for recognition have annually eliminated the equivalent of 75,000 tons of air pollutants, 1,325 tons of water pollutants, 500 million gallons of polluted wastewater, and 2,900 tons of sludge per year. In addition, 3M and scores of other companies have developed ways to recover wastes that are used either internally or sold for a profit. Based on a 1977 survey of industry, the Census Bureau estimated the value of the energy and materials recovered as a result of pollution control measures to be more than $950 million. Similar results are occurring abroad. A study of Great Britain concluded, "It is clear that resource conservation and pollution control are complementary, and that much of the cost of the latter is paid for by the former."[15]

Transforming wastes into profitable resources has been stimulated in recent years through the establishment of waste bourses

(exchanges). Basically, the bourse brings a company with an industrial waste into contact with another company that can profitably use the waste. Wastes that might be a liability because of high disposal costs or possible damage to the environment can give the seller additional income and the buyer a cheaper source of raw material. The United States generates an estimated 344 million metric (wet) tons of industrial waste each year. If only 10 percent of this waste could be utilized or recycled, waste exchanges would prove their worth. Cooperation between exchanges and the best ways to reach small and medium-sized industries must be explored further.

One corporate practice that leads to significant resource savings and does not involve wastes is materials substitution. In many cases, the driving force of materials substitution is the development of technology. Communications is a prime example, for technological developments have significantly reduced materials requirements through solid-state electronics, microfilms, microwave transmission, and commercial satellites. Finding a completely new way to perform the function of a component or system is known as functional or system substitution. The transistor, for instance, requires perhaps one-millionth of the material needed to make the vacuum tube it replaces.

An Expanded Role in the Future Although corporations have already undertaken significant resource conservation activities, there is potential for considerably more, particularly regarding recycling, energy conservation, and pollution control process change.

Although recycling rates for a number of materials are fairly high, they have remained on a plateau for over a decade. Despite highly publicized programs to increase aluminum recycling, the market share for recycled aluminum as a percentage of the nation's total metal consumption still stands at 20 percent, the same ratio as in 1964. Over the same period, copper has remained virtually static, lead and zinc are both down about 2 percent, and tin has fallen from a 29 percent market share to 20 percent. Thus, even for a relatively high-valued commodity like copper, we are losing 40 percent of the supply available for recycling.

These ratios are likely to increase substantially in the 1980s due to the increasingly favorable economics of recycling. Recycled materials have a financial edge, since they are closer in composition to the final product than are primary raw materials. Gone are the costly mining, milling, and processing of ores, as well as much of the waste and pollution associated with production. Also, recycling can be carried out in plants that are simpler and so require less capital investment. This production is also more flexible because recycling plants can be constructed in much less time than new mining and smelting facilities, 29

and they can be located where they are most convenient. The operating costs of recycling plants are lower than primary production facilities, in some case by as much as 65 to 75 percent. A large part of these savings are energy savings.

As favorable as these points are, business may still not undertake the socially optimum degree of recycling because of various government-induced hinderances. The actions that government should take to foster recycling are discussed below. Industry itself should explore the concept of reverse distribution channels for recycling.[16] In these channels, producers of recyclable and reusable solid waste material are conventional consumers, and the final users of these materials are traditional producers. Manufacturers, therefore, must go beyond classic concepts of marketing and look toward consumers not only as potential buyers, but also as potential raw material sources. The reverse channel of distribution must become highly efficient and sophisticated, designed to accumulate and sort out recyclable materials and make them economically available to producers.

Energy conservation efforts have just scratched the surface. In building construction, technical improvements can save 50 percent or more in office buildings and 80 percent or more in some new houses. Because the potential savings from insulation and other energy conservation measures in the home are so large, public utilities should lend money to its customers for these purposes. The customers would have lower energy bills, allowing them to pay their normal utility rate while paying off the debt without feeling much strain. When the debt is paid off, they would reap the fuel savings while the utility would have earned interest on its loan and spent less to gain the same amount of energy.

"Cogeneration," the generating of electricity as a by-product of the process steam produced in industry, is another area of great potential. According to a study directed by Paul McCracken, by 1985 U.S. industry could meet approximately half its own electricity needs by this means, compared to about a seventh in 1977.[17] This rate of cogeneration would save fuel equivalent to 2 to 3 million barrels of oil per day as well as investments of $20 to $50 billion.

Reduction of per capita consumption of packaging materials through improved packaging techniques would save energy by reducing the solid waste load and by reducing the amount of packaging material produced. Potential total energy savings are estimated to be 0.6 quad/year, approximately six times the energy required for landfilling municipal solid waste in the United States.[18]

Most conservation measures to date have been applied to existing structures or equipment. The introduction of new facilities holds the greatest potential. To gauge the potential, Thomas Long and Lee Schipper examined production facilities in Europe, particularly West

Germany and Holland, and in Japan, where industrial plants incorporate numerous technological advances over the older U.S. capital stock.[19] Energy requirements for production of primary aluminum, cement, and polyvinylchloride (PVC) in these countries led them to conclude that new capital facilities can and will substitute for energy. Thus, they postulate a "new cycle of capital investment" in the United States stemming from the energy price rises. In a 1978 survey, corporate officials predicted that replacement of entire plants or offices with more energy-efficient ones, while only a small part of spending so far, would be a significant factor in capital outlays a few years hence.[20]

To date, only a small fraction of corporations have undertaken process change to control (or prevent) pollution. Since the pioneers in this area have experienced such significant economic and/or energy savings, it seems inevitable that market forces alone will dictate the expansion of this resource-conserving pollution control method.

As a general principle, corporations in the future are going to have to learn how to get more from less and then have the will to do it. They will have to place greater emphasis on the development of production methods, technologies, and products that extend the life of nonrenewable resources; maximize the sustainable yield of renewable resources; reduce energy and resource use per unit of output; eliminate or cut down on the creation of waste; allow for recycling; provide for greater longevity and durability; and ensure that they do not overburden the "public service" functions (such as waste assimilation) rendered by the natural environment.

Since many of these are design problems, corporations must launch a design revolution that will improve the performance (basically energy efficiency) and durability of consumer goods. Products designed to be durable, to use less materials, to be easily repaired, to pollute less, and to have lower operating costs will suddenly be recognized for their value—their life-cycle costs will be lower than competing, less efficient brands. Design possibilities include the use of corrosion-resistant materials, replacement of rubber belts with gears, the sealing of sensitive parts, modular construction for easy repair, and updating and synergetic (doing more with less) innovations. A related design problem is to make a product easily recyclable by having parts that are readily separable.

Specifically, in the 1980s corporations must adopt an environmentally oriented mode of industrial project planning, one in which inputs and means related to environmental concerns, values, processes, conditions, and interrelationships are continuously and carefully taken into account during planning. Since the object of environmentally oriented planning is the avoidance, or at least the minimization, or adverse environmental consequences, the range of

possible actions include plant locations, input mixes, construction methods, scales of activity, process technologies, transport systems, and output patterns. The question, "What impact would this action have on the environment?" must be asked and answered throughout the course of planning.

Viewed most broadly, environmentally sound planning can yield economic, political, and technical payoffs that include the avoidance of delays, smoother relations with the public and government agencies, better protection against spurious allegations, improved public image, and the development of expertise that can be sold to other companies. Thus, environmental, energy, and economic interests converge to put a premium on greater and greater efficiency in the industrial process—a new efficiency that can, at one and same time, cut costs, conserve energy, and curb pollution.

THE ROLE OF GOVERNMENT

The government's one-resource-at-a-time approach to natural resource problems continues to have serious adverse effects. The "national" policy has really "emerged" as the result of an accretion of numerous individual decisions. This after-the-fact policy takes on some of the contradictions accumulated over separate and disparate decisions. By continuing its present piecemeal materials policy, the government is increasing the likelihood of inducing shortages or prolonging those caused by natural or political events, here and abroad.

Economists must share some of the blame for this rather lax attitude toward resources and their future availability. In the past, they have not included preservation of the resource base in their list of macroeconomic goals needing explicit policy measures. They have relied on the invisible hand of the market to match new technology against depletion. But now, as material flows are becoming enormously larger, lead times shorter, and the environmental and technological effects more pervasive, it is time to make preservation of the resource base an explicit policy issue. Since the resource base is shared intergenerationally, certain questions must be explicitly addressed, which even perfect markets could not answer: Will it be shared fairly? In its use of materials, how can the economy be kept from drifting into unlivable futures?

What is needed in the United States are a comprehensive analysis of material supply and demand over the foreseeable future and the formulation of a national materials policy developed as a joint effort by government, business, and the public interest groups. This national policy should be designed to provide adequate resources and resource substitutes for the future, stressing conservation measures, while

balancing material needs and environmental considerations. The

government's role in fostering various forms of conservation is discussed below.

Potential
Conservation Policies
Government must establish, as a central element of a comprehensive natural resources policy, economic incentives to turn our industrial structure toward less resource- and energy-intensive technologies and production processes. Recycling is perhaps the area where national policy could have the most significant impact.

The first issue to consider is, Why should the federal government concern itself with recycling? There are four major benefits from increased recycling that are in the long-run national interest. First, recycling the material in postconsumer waste will help reduce the increasing demands on the world's virgin resources, which are making their extraction more and more costly in terms of capital requirements and environmental degradation. Second, it will provide a domestic source of materials that will reduce the political uncertainties of foreign sources of supply and the adverse impact of the demand for imported materials on the nation's balance of trade. Third, it will provide a smaller waste stream that has more manageable constituent parts, alleviating a major, costly problem for cities. Finally, the production of manufactured products from recycled materials will generally result in a significant saving of energy.

The energy-saving feature is potentially very important, since one-fifth of the total U.S. energy budget is now spent on materials production. Maximum savings from recycling 100 percent scrap would reduce energy output 47 percent for steel, 96 percent for aluminum, and approximately 90 percent for copper. Looking more closely at steel, even the limited use of scrap by the industry in 1976 saved 14 million tons of coal and the equivalent of 5.7 billion gallons of gasoline. Moreover, when steel mills use ferrous scrap in lieu of iron ore, there is an 86 percent reduction in air pollution, a 76 percent reduction in water pollution, and a 40 percent reduction in water use.[21] Despite such significant benefits, the government subsidizes the use of iron ore with a 13 percent depletion allowance and by permitting railroad freight charges that are three times as high for scrap as for iron ore.

Because all other countries still depend largely on conventional sources for the supply of natural resources, a U.S. commitment toward an economically maximum recycling technology would establish it as the leader in this field and result in American stewardship over an approaching worldwide industry.

Three categories of problems tend to inhibit the recycling of materials: the lack of adequate technology; economic and institutional issues; and problems of information and interpretation. Many of the technical processing problems have a common origin in contamina-

tion, which typically characterizes secondary materials. The economic problem revolves around the fact that secondary materials often serve in a substitutional capacity. During periods of high demand, they are used to fill gaps in supply, but they are first to feel the effects of reduced demand. Thus, the prices of many secondary materials are more volatile than those of their primary counterparts, which represents a substantial deterrent to investment in recycling. There are also artificial barriers and disincentives to recycling, such as freight rates and taxation that discriminate in favor of primary production. Finally, we lack reliable information on the magnitude of the pools of the major secondary materials, so that we cannot determine the physically possible maximum production from secondary sources.

There are a number of specific steps government could take to correct these problems, particularly the economic and institutional ones. It took one step in the National Energy Act of 1978 by establishing a 10 percent tax credit on recycling equipment and setting goals for increasing the use of recycled commodities. This initiative was important in that it was the federal government's first demonstration of a willingness to provide a viable means for industry to increase the recycling of solid waste materials. It does not, however, get at the root, structural problems that would necessitate broad-ranging government reform.

First, government must ensure that price reflects scarcity value and that economic neutrality is achieved as far as the production and use of primary (virgin) and secondary (recycled) materials are concerned. Ending freight rates that discriminate against secondary materials would be a minimal first step to encourage conservation of scarce resources and to provide appropriate signals for the marketplace to reflect true scarcity values.

A more fundamental initiative would be for government to repeal the percentage depletion allowance for minerals, a provision of the tax code that encourages consumption of virgin over recycled materials. This tax preference undermines long-term stable demand for recycled materials and, thus, is a major deterrent to utilization of resources in postconsumer waste. Percentage depletion has encouraged the growth of large, vertically integrated materials companies that shelter their income by maintaining high prices for their virgin material input and allocating their profits to virgin material production. These companies are structured, both physically and institutionally, to use wholly owned virgin materials as their primary feed. They purchase postconsumer scrap only to respond to peaks in the demand for their product; their demand for recycled material fluctuates accordingly. In the steel industry, the effect of tax preferences more than accounts for the difference between the cost of producing a ton of steel from scrap
34 and the lower cost of producing it from virgin material.

Although the evidence supporting the argument that the repeal of tax subsidies will increase the rate of recycling is incomplete, the evidence to support their continuation is even weaker. Nor should new tax subsidies for the consumption of recycled materials be created. Given that tax subsidies for virgin material consumption are an inefficient means of expanding the supply of minerals, there is no reason to suppose that a tax credit for the purchase of recycled materials would be a more efficient expenditure of tax dollars.

Also in the tax area, there is a problem with the definition of taxation categories. Depending on the specific technology employed, some recycling or resource recovery plants can be classified as engaged in a "manufacturing or processing function" or in "mining," whereas some others are neither. This means that some recycling industries may not qualify for existing tax incentives offered to manufacturing: accelerated depreciation periods for capital investments, as well as current income tax rates that are frequently lower than otherwise.

Government should also take steps to internalize the cost of disposing of materials. Presently, governments discourage the recycling of containers and paper products by assessing the cost of discarding such materials against general revenues rather than against the price of the containers and paper products. To remedy this, the government could impose a schedule of national solid waste disposal charges on the sale or transfer, at the bulk production level, of rigid consumer containers and of flexible consumer packaging and paper. This could double present rates of paper recycling, a very considerable savings since packaging and paper products make up (by weight) almost one-half of the total waste stream and 80 percent of all product-type wastes. The government could also review the experience of the French, Japanese, and Norwegian governments in setting up orderly guaranteed markets for recycled paper through such measures as subsidized collecting centers, storage space, and guaranteed prices. A mandatory deposit on carbonated beverage containers would also internalize external costs. Studies show that such a system in 1976 would have saved 150–200 billion Btu per year and about 13 billion pounds of raw materials. Sweden recently established a similar mandatory deposit system for automobiles. A tax of SwKr 300 is levied at time of purchase and is refundable when the car is turned into a scrap yard. Since the company passes the cost on to the buyer, since no competitive differentials between companies arise, and since the money is finally returned, this procedure should rate "supportive" to all concerned.

One form of recycling that deserves special consideration by the federal government is the recycling of urban solid wastes. The annual disposal cost in the late 1970s for approximately 144 million tons per year of municipal postconsumer solid waste was about $4 billion.   *35*

Although the recovery and reuse of these discarded materials would significantly reduce these disposal costs, the current recovery rate is estimated at only 6 to 7 percent. A recovery rate is technically achievable, though not yet fully price competitive, that would provide about 40 percent of the metal, glass, plastics, fibers, and rubber needed each year by manufacturing industries. The institutional separation of energy generation by public utilities and waste disposal by municipalities must be seriously questioned from both an economic and energy perspective. In 1978 the United States recovered only 1 percent of the energy potential of municipal solid waste, while Denmark, which integrates the two functions, recovered 60 percent. The energy recovery potential from our municipal solid waste load in 1978 was equivalent to 400,000 barrels of oil per day.

Mining this "urban ore" has begun. In 1979, five refuse-to-energy plants processing more than 500 tons daily were in operation. Industry experts expect that within seven years about 17 percent of the nation's garbage will be recovered in 20 large plants and 50 small ones (treating less than 500 tons daily). In addition, Harrisburg, Pa., and Duluth, Minn., are the first cities in the United States to adopt co-disposal, a technique pioneered in Europe for simultaneously disposing of garbage and sludge. In Duluth, the thermal co-disposal plant will conserve three million gallons of oil costing $1 million per year, will conserve an estimated 1,000 acres of land during the next 20 years, and will reclaim 14 to 25 tons per day of ferrous metals to be sold at $35 per ton.[22]

The federal government could facilitate further movement in this direction by making grants to competing municipalities to help them experiment with ways to switch from solid waste disposal to resource recovery in the manner most suited to their individual community needs. Such grants are essential because before cities can justify making capital expenditures, they have to first figure out how to overcome the technical, marketing, financial, legal, and organizational barriers. Thus, the initial 63 resource recovery planning grants that EPA awarded in 1979 should be carefully evaluated and, if proven effective, new ones should be made available.

Also in the solid waste area, the federal government could consider eliminating its disincentives, in the form of tax and revenue-sharing policies, that by providing financial support have prevented communities and citizens from giving serious consideration to the adoption of local user fees for financing solid waste management. This would allow communities to make an unbiased decision about the economic and social merits of having citizens pay for that proportion of the municipal disposal services that they actually use. Quantity-based local user fees have the potential to stimulate both a reduction in the quantity of waste individuals put out for collection and disposal

and an increase in source separation and resource recovery. In addition to providing a more equitable means of payment for waste collection and disposal than the current flat fee and local tax-financed systems, local user fees would also heighten citizen consciousness about both waste and resource recovery.

Although recycling is an essential feature of the conserver society, it nevertheless consumes energy and often causes severe pollution problems. Also, the question of the optimum amount of recycling has different answers for different materials at different times, depending on the labor, capital, indirect materials, and energy required for recycling. The economic optimum for recycling is also affected by other materials conservation strategies such as the increased durability of products or substitutions in the materials from which they are made. The effects of such changes are not yet well understood. All of these uncertainties support the view that recycling is one element in a complex materials supply system, and they point to the importance of a systems approach to materials conservation.

An important additional goal, therefore, is to increase the effective life of manufactured products, i.e., to promote reuse rather than recycling. Although providing effective rewards for the manufacture of durable products is difficult, the government could consider a number of simple steps: setting mandatory minimum standards for durability, requiring the labeling of guaranteed and expected lifetime, requiring corporations to provide consumer information on lifetime costs and, in some cases, testing by government agencies (analogous to existing tests for automobile fuel economy). Because automobiles impose such substantial costs in terms of depleted resources and pollution, mandatory minimum standards for durability and sustained performance (including at least the engine and drive train) should be considered, backed by a federal testing and consumer information program.

In general, the free market imperfection of consumer choices based on insufficient or misleading information should be reduced by a vigorous government effort to ensure accurate advertising and full labeling of products. Full labeling would include giving consumers the life-cycle cost of the product, which can be presented as the average cost per year of buying and keeping a product in good repair over its life span. Once everything is priced on this basis, a revolution will take place in the manufacturing industry. Manufacturers will benefit not only when they can keep their costs down but also when they can keep their customers' costs down. The government could also choose, in certain instances, to influence consumer choice by altering the cost of energy or resource-intensive goods or activities; for example, imposing an excise tax on gas-guzzling cars. Or it could provide the public with alternative services that effectively reduce demand for energy and raw

materials; for example, mass transit is a public investment that helps reduce reliance on imported oil.

A Long-Run, Integrated Policy Framework

We have become great in a material sense because of the lavish use of our resources, and we have just reason to be proud of our growth. But the time has come to inquire seriously what will happen when our forests are gone, when the coal, the iron, the oil, and the gas are exhausted, when the soils shall have been still further impoverished and washed into the streams, polluting the rivers, denuding the fields, and obstructing navigation. These questions do not relate only to the next century or to the next generation. One distinguishing characteristic of really civilized men is foresight; we have to, as a nation, exercise foresight for this nation in the future.[23]

These were the words of Theodore Roosevelt in 1911 in his keynote address to a White House Conference on the Conservation of Natural Resources. Unfortunately, the nation has not heeded his advice. Indeed, much of the malaise afflicting Americans is due to their perception that the United States is walking backward into the future. With no vision of what America could or should be like in the future, the nation drifts into an uncertain future like a ship without a compass or even a clear destination. It is little wonder that Americans today keenly sense that their government leaders do not have a good idea of "whither we are tending."

Key federal decision makers continue to view trends as isolated phenomena, even though it is the mode of interaction among the major forces and trends influencing long-term growth that is usually critical in determining their ultimate impact. Tackling problems on such a piecemeal basis leads to policy "solutions" that are too narrowly based and often produce results favorable in one area but counterproductive in another. For example, an environmental policy, an energy policy, and an urban policy may each be perfectly reasonable when judged on their individual merits, but may culminate in an untenable or disastrous whole.

The traditional institutions of national government are, simply put, badly designed for the kinds of problems they now face. They tend to be bounded by the artificial frontiers that survive from the history of rational thought (physics, biology, economics), from the history of government activity in simpler times (mining, merchant marine, forestry, the regulation of commerce), and from the historic professions (law, medicine, engineering)—while the real world agenda consists mostly of interdisciplinary, interdepartmental, and interprofessional problems. Government agencies are basically not organized to handle the problems that cut across disciplines, specialties, and bureaucracies; to heighten awareness of the interconnectedness of

things; and to encourage integrative training, staff work, and decision making.

Also complicating the policy framework is the internationalization of what used to be considered national decision making. Three categories of problems that no longer fit into national policy frameworks can be identified. First, there are the inherently global environments, where the issues that arise are unmanageable except in a global context. Familiar examples are the management of ocean resources; pollution of, and traffic through, the atmosphere and the oceans; the human uses of outer space; the protection of the ozone layer; and weather reporting, forecasting, and large-scale modification. Second, there are issues of global concern because they involve the integrity of crucial physical resources and systems shared by the human race: soils and fresh water systems; the basic ecological systems that make fisheries, forests, cropland, and pastureland possible; and such global natural cycles and budgets as heat, water, and energy. In a third category are issues of global interest because the impact of what happens in one area reverberates in all. Examples are the policies of governments on population control, and the condition of natural and manmade habitats; national decisions that affect such irreplaceable supports of individual and social life as food and energy supplies; the violation of what have come to be regarded as universal human rights; and the prevalence of human poverty, which is to say the failure to meet what have come to be regarded as entitlements to basic human needs.

Global problems, technologies, concerns, and interests do not necessitate global government. National governments will still be the basic building blocks of world order. They will, however, increasingly find themselves having to collaborate to get things done that simply cannot be done by translating "independence" into "isolation."

The fact that the really critical issues before the country are not the immediate and isolated ones but the interrelated and long-range ones suggests the desirability of developing a new policy framework that would examine these interrelationships and be anticipatory in nature. However, policy formulation cannot be forward-looking until clear national goals and priorities have been established, to which policies can be directed and measurement to assess progress applied. If government policies are going to effectively govern the long-run forces influencing growth, rather than be governed by them, a national growth policy framework will be to be developed that would fulfill three functions:

■ Establishing national priorities and goals and measuring progress toward achieving the goals
■ Conducting on-going analysis of long-range trends influencing the   *39*

socioeconomic system, and anticipating problems likely to arise
■ Guiding the coordination and integration of policies

Comprehensiveness will be the key to the success of a national growth policy process. It will have to provide for harmonizing frequently conflicting aims within our broader social and environmental, as well as purely economic, objectives. In particular, environmental policy should be more closely coordinated with both energy policy and housing and urban development policy.

Since intensive use of energy and raw materials is accompanied by potentially high pollution loads, gains in environmental quality could be achieved by coordinating energy and raw materials policy with environmental policy. Such policy coordination, in the context of a conserver society goal, could entail such measures as the recovery of raw materials waste and use of waste heat; lengthening product lives; and substituting low "throughput" processes or products for high users of energy and raw materials. Policy coordination should also ensure that the environmental costs of alternative choices among energy and raw material sources are reflected in public and private decisions.

Urban policies, developed to make cities more pleasant and more efficient in providing resources, can be given a strong environmental component. In addition to aiming at significantly reduced pollution loads, amenity production should be an important environmental objective. Renovation of old houses and buildings is a key element. It is not necessarily more costly and its resource content is different: it utilizes more labor, less energy, fewer raw materials, and less capital.

EPA has taken, and continues to take, many steps to help distressed cities. But there is a clear need for better coordination between EPA and other federal agencies. For example, firmer links between EPA's regulatory functions and the varied federal credit programs will facilitate achievement of environmental objectives without heavy social and economic costs. Similarly, stronger ties between EPA and the Department of Transportation will permit consideration of transportation options simultaneously respond to local air quality, land use, and development priorities.

Finally, growth policy process must not be allowed to operate in a domestic vacuum. Interdependence, a hard reality, demands closer international cooperation in economic policies. Energy—or Eurodollars or multinational corporations—is not alone in creating problems beyond the capacity of any nation to resolve; inflation, worker migration patterns, pollution, and scores of other issues have also taken on transnational dimensions. Because of this, government "drift" must be replaced by purposive, coordinated policies and action. As Winston Churchill stressed, "Those who are possessed of a definite body of doctrine and of deeply rooted convictions upon it will be in a

much better position to deal with the shifts and surprises of daily affairs than those who are merely taking short views, and indulging their natural impulses as they are evoked by what they read from day to day."[24] A national growth policy in the United States in the 1980s could be influenced by the doctrine of qualitative growth, a major element of which would be the conserver society goal.

Granted, the process of developing a national growth policy that is integrative, anticipatory, and goal suggesting is much more of an art form than a science. Some may, on that basis, question its validity. To them, Lord Keynes gently suggests, "There will be no harm in making mild preparations for our destiny."

There should be no illusions that a national growth policy will solve all current problems or prevent major ones from arising in the future. It will, however, help us regain our confidence in our ability to manage our affairs, to deal with our problems, and to take charge of our future. Most importantly, it should help bring about a renewed sense of national unity and purpose.

FOOTNOTES TO CHAPTER 2

1. Daniel Yankelovich and Bernard Lefkowitz, "Public Debate on Growth: Preparing for Resolution," paper presented at Third Biennial Woodlands Conference on Growth Policy, October 27, 1979, p. 1.

2. E. F. Schumacher, *Small is Beautiful,* New York: Harper Torchbooks, 1973.

3. Talbot Page, *Conservation and Economic Efficiency,* Baltimore: Johns Hopkins University Press, 1977, p. 4.

4. Sam H. Schurr and Joel Darmstadter, "The Energy Connection," *Resources,* Fall 1976, pp. 1-2, 5-7.

5. Joel Darmstadter, Joy Dunkerly, and Jack Alterman, "International Variations in Energy Use: Findings from a Comparative Study," *Annual Reveiw of Energy,* 1978, pp. 201-24.

6. John G. Myers, "Energy Conservation and Economic Growth—Are They Incompatible?" *The Conference Board Record,* July 1976; Institute for Energy Analysis, *U.S. Energy and Economic Growth, 1975-2010,* September 1976; Dale Jorgenson, "The Economic Impact of Policies to Reduce U.S. Energy Growth," Harvard Institute of Economic Research Discussion Paper #644, August 1978; William Nordhaus, "What is the Tradeoff Between Energy Consumption and Real Income?" unpublished paper, Yale University, 1977.

7. *Science, Technology and Society—A Prospective Look,* Washington, D.C. : National Academy of Sciences, p. 16.

8. Science Council of Canada, Natural Resource Policy Issues in Canada, Ottawa: Minister of Supply and Services, January 1973, p. 39.

9. Cited in Science Council of Canada, *Canada as a Conserver Society,* Ottawa, Minister of Supply and Services, September 1977, p. 14.

10. Yankelovich and Lefkowitz, op. cit.

11. *New York Times Magazine,* September 12, 1970.

12. Louis Lundborg, *Future Without Shock,* New York: W. W. Norton, 1974, p. 84.

13. Ibid.

14. *Business Week,* February 1978.

15. J. F. Lowe and M. H. Atkins, "Resource Conservation and Environmental Control," *Resources Policy,* March 1978, p. 81.

16. Peter M. Ginter and Jack M. Starling, "Reverse Distribution Channels for Recycling," *California Management Review,* Spring 1978.

17. Paul McCracken et. al., *Industrial Energy Center Study,* report to NSF, PB 243824, National Technical Information Service, June 1975.

18. R. W. Serth and R. S. Hockett, *Energy Requirements of Present Pollution Control Technology,* EPA Report 600/7-78-084, May 1978.

19. Thomas Long and Lee Schipper, "Resources and Energy Substitution," in Volume 4 *Resources and Energy* of Joint Economic Committee study series *U.S. Economic Growth from 1976–1986: Prospects Problems and Patterns,* Washington D.C., Government Printing Ofice, November 16, 1976.

20. Cited in Ralph Winter, "Firms Spend Millions to Cut Use of Energy," *Wall Street Journal,* February 9, 1978, p. 1.

21. The above figures were quoted in "Fighting Over Scraps: Steel Mills vs. Recyclers," *Washington Post,* September 4, 1977.

22. Betsy Goggin and Michele Hodak, "Co-Disposal: A New Technology," *EPA Journal,* September 1979, pp. 20–1.

23. Quoted in Roderick Nash, *The American Environment: Readings in the History of Conservation,* Menlo Park, California: Addison-Wesley, 1968, p. 50.

24. Winston S. Churchill, *The Gathering Storm,* Boston: Houghton-Mifflin, 1948, p. 210.

3

THE BENEFITS OF ENVIRONMENTAL REGULATION

In the past few years, government regulations have been indicted for a host of evils. Particularly important is the charge that they forced "nonproductive" expenditures on industry, thus contributing to the productivity decline in the 1970s and to the high inflation rates that still prevail. The assumption implicit in such arguments is that compliance expenditures are not worth it—that the costs are greater than the benefits.

In part, this assumption stems from the ready availability of cost figures and the difficulty of assessing benefits. Certainly, there can be no disguising the fact that pollution control measures have been quite costly. It is estimated that in 1978 total pollution control costs in the United States were $46.7 billion. A little over half of this total was spent in response to federal environmental legislation; the rest would have been spent without it and includes activities such as trash disposal. Businesses' capital investment for pollution control was about $7.1 billion, 4.7 percent of their total plant and equipment investment.

The critical question, which should form the heart of the debate over the impact of regulations on economic activity, is: Is society getting its money's worth? If the popular implicit assumption that the costs exceed the benefits is correct, the regulations should indeed be scaled back or made more cost-effective. If, on the other hand, the positive effects generated by environmental regulations—their benefits—are more highly valued than the economic burden they impose on us, the compliance expenditures are good economic investments.

There are few quantitative estimates of the benefits. Yet those that have been done (highlighted below) conclude that, to date, the benefits have exceeded the costs. This is the case even though the analyses are only partial, excluding many benefits that cannot be easily quantified. Thus, the traditional benefits study offers too narrow a perspective.

The purpose of this chapter is to offer a broad perspective on benefits. In addition to those benefits that can be quantified through traditional economic analysis, there are three main types of benefits that must also be considered to get the complete picture of the effects of environmental regulations: the improvement that has taken place in environmental quality; the positive impacts on such economic variables as GNP, employment, and even prices; and the stimulus to industrial innovation provided by regulations.

TRADITIONAL STUDIES OF BENEFITS

Services Provided by the Environment

In economic analysis, the economist normally views the environment from a different perspective than an environmentalist does. The quality of the air mantle is not important in and of itself but because it has, among other things, direct mortality and morbidity effects on people. Thus, as a first step, an economic definition of the environment makes man the measure of all things. A further refinement views the environment as a nonreproducible capital asset which, over time, yields a stream of services for man.

The most basic services provided by the environment involve the support of human life. These services are threatened, and in many cases reduced in volume, as a second class of services—the dispersing, storing, and assimilating of residuals that are generated as a by-product of economic activity—increases over time. Amenity services, a third class, primarily encompasses the pursuit of recreational activities. Finally, the environment serves as a source of material inputs to the economy. As with life support and amenity services, these material input flows can also be impaired in quality and quantity by increases in the flow of residuals absorptive services.

Environmental quality can thus be defined as the level and composition of the stream of all environmental services except waste receptor services. In economic terms, the ultimate measure of environmental quality is the value that people place on these services. This willingness to pay constitutes the "benefits" of environmental quality, even though many of the services comprising environmental quality do not pass through markets and, hence, do not have prices attached to them. Nevertheless, this nonmonetary income is as much a part of people's real income or welfare as their willingness to pay for marketable goods and services.

Operating in the same economics framework, the damage induced by pollution is equal to the reduction in the value of environmental quality caused by the disposal of residuals. As such, environmental damage conforms to the classical economic notion of opportunity costs.

Empirical Estimates from Air Pollution Studies

Cost-benefit analyses usually follow a sequence of basic steps: (1) enumerating the effects of a proposed action; (2) classifying each effect as either a cost or benefit; (3) relating each effect quantitatively to the scope of the proposed action; (4) translating each effect into a common metric and common time period; and (5) judging the proposed action by comparing the costs and benefits. The third step is perhaps the greatest

stumbling block, for there is no universal agreement on either the extent to which human health is adversely affected by air pollution or the exact association between exposure and ill effects (the dose-response relationship) or on which specific pollutants are the most pernicious.

There have been more studies of the benefits from air pollution control than from water pollution control. Those that do exist on the latter deal primarily with recreational opportunities foregone, and they yield few empirical estimates. The more voluminous air pollution analyses reflect the fact that the damage associated with air pollution is more diverse. It includes the costs associated with damage to human health, the costs of pollution-related cleaning and maintenance activities, the costs of inhibited growth and destruction of plant life, and the reductions in property values associated with air pollution. Studies that have tried to estimate the economic value of the first and last of these effects will be discussed.

Lester Lave has conducted extensive studies of the health-related benefits from air pollution controls. After taking account of the extreme difficulties in measuring health-related damages from air pollution, in 1970 Lave and his associates estimated the relationship between mortality rates and various measures of the dimensions of air pollution levels.[1] They concluded that pollution is a significant explanatory variable for death rates in all age categories, although the effects do vary by age category and the measure of pollution used. Specifically, they estimated that abating pollution by 50 percent would be worth about $2 billion per year in terms of the economic benefits of increased days worked and decreased health expenditures.

In 1977 Lave and Eugene Seskin coauthored the book *Air Pollution and Human Health,* which provided more updated estimates. They concluded that there are statistical links between some air pollutants and human illness:

> In the largest U.S. cities, there are close relationships between the mortality rate and air pollution (as measured by sulfates, sulphur dioxide, suspended particulates and possibly a nitrogen compound, such as nitric oxide). The air pollutants for which we failed to find consistent, statistically significant time-series relationships with mortality rates were nitrates, nitrogen dioxide, carbon monoxide and hydrocarbons.[2]

Specifically, they estimated that if legally required abatements from 1971 smokestack pollution levels of 88 percent in sulfates and 58 percent in particulates were achieved in 1979, the benefits in terms of improved health alone would be $16.1 billion (in 1973 dollars), a figure more than 70 percent greater than the EPA estimated $9.5 billion (1973

dollars) annual abatement cost.

Substantial work in estimating the adverse economic effects of air pollution has been undertaken by relating air pollution levels to property values. This approach is based upon the belief that the rents for property capture the bulk of adverse effects from air pollution, including health effects.

The first such study was done by Ridker and his associates in the mid-1960s.[3] In their study of the St. Louis metropolitan area, they found that air pollution levels, especially sulfation, were significant explanatory variables concerning property values. Due to high sulfation levels, they estimated an annual loss for the entire St. Louis area of almost $5 million.

In 1971, Crocker studied the relationship between air pollution and property values for the city of Chicago, employing data on each of 1,288 single family residential property transactions from 1964-67.[4] He found that the annual damages from modest additional amounts of particulates and sulphur dioxide ranged from about $350 to $600 per household.

Crocker also served as the project director for a study released in March 1979 that, at the time, represented the state of the art in benefits analysis.[5] It encompassed both the health and property value effects. Since it is the most comprehensive study to date, it will be examined in detail.

The study emphasized two areas. First, the analytical and empirical methods of economics were used to develop hypotheses on disease etiologies and to value labor productivity and consumer losses due to air pollution-induced mortality and morbidity. Second, new experimental techniques for measuring the value of air quality improvements and other environmental amenities were developed and tested for a specific area, the South Coast Air Basin of southern California.

The research team developed two approaches for determining health effects and valuing them in economic terms. First, economic losses were approximated when a dose-response relationship was known between mortality rates and air pollution, or between days lost from work due to illness (productivity loss) and air pollution. Their second approach was an attempt to observe the direct effect of air pollution on economic factors, thus avoiding the necessity of developing dose-response relationships. The object of this approach, based on traditional microeconomic theory, was to derive consumer willingness to pay to avoid illness by developing relationships employing data on wages, wealth, and socioeconomic and health status characteristics as well as pollution exposures.

With regard to the first approach, they used a data set on 60 U.S.
cities to estimate a human dose-response expression in which 1970 city-

wide mortality rates for major disease categories were statistically associated with various population characteristics. Multiplying the population at risk (150 million) by the assumed value of safety ($340,000 lower-bound and $1,000,000 upper-bound estimates) and then by the average reduction in risk gave a crude approximation of the benefits for a 60 percent reduction in national urban ambient concentrations of particulates and sulfur dioxide, respectively. The resulting figures were $5.1 to $15.9, "an order of magnitude smaller than other estimates."

The morbidity approach employed data on the health and the time and budget allocations of a random sampling of the civilian population nationwide. They found that for most of the dose-response expressions, air pollution appeared to be significantly associated with increased acute or chronic illness. Air pollution-induced chronic illness caused a much larger decline in labor productivity than air pollution-induced acute illness. Applying a 60 percent reduction in the 1970 air pollution level to the 1977 total population yielded an increase in value of urban labor productivity of $36.4 billion (in 1978 dollars). With the caveat that the magnitude is extremely sensitive to the underlying assumptions, the authors concluded that "the economic gains from the morbidity reduction effects of air pollution control may have been greatly undervalued, perhaps because most prior research efforts have concentrated upon mortality rather than morbidity."[6]

Combining the mortality and morbidity figures yields a total benefits figure of $41.5 billion. Since the actual reduction in particulates from 1970 to 1977 was only 12 percent or one-fifth of the study's 60 percent assumption, the annual benefits are $8.3 billion, which significantly exceeds the $6.7 billion the nation was spending in 1977 to control all pollutants from stationary sources.

In the property value part of the study, two rather distinct approaches to valuation of environmental quality were employed: (1) an analysis to determine how some actual market prices, such as real property prices, are influenced by environmental quality attributes, and (2) a survey technique to induce individuals to reveal their actual preferences, in monetary terms, for environmental attributes.

Under the first approach, the researchers found that a 30 percent improvement in air quality would produce annual benefits of $500 per household or $950 million in aggregate due to increased real estate values. The interview approach found that Los Angeles area residents were willing to pay $650 per household or $650 million in total per year for a 30 percent improvement. Thus, rather than overestimating the value of cleaner air and better visibility, people were paying more for it than they said they would be willing to pay.

Acknowledging that their estimates could not be considered "highly accurate," the research team nevertheless felt that the study provided

three benchmarks:

1. Many benefits traditionally viewed as intangible and thereby nonmeasureable can, in fact, be measured and made comparable to economic value as expressed in markets.
2. Aesthetic experiences and morbidity (illness) effects may dominate the measure of benefits, as opposed to previous emphasis on mortality health effects.
3. The likely economic benefits of air quality improvements are perhaps as much as an order of magnitude greater than previous studies had hypothesized.[7]

Shortcomings of Benefit Studies

Having come through the pangs of birth and infancy, benefit analysis is now entering the awkward toddler's stage. There is a clear destination in mind, but the means to get there are still uncertain. Excellent critiques of benefits analysis have been offered by environmental economists Edwin H. Clark II and Robert Haveman.

Clark, focusing on the regulatory arena and acknowledging that there is little dispute about the need for identifying what benefits a regulation is expected to produce, emphasizes that attempting elaborate, monetized benefit estimation will be very expensive and increase uncertainty, and may decrease information and be biased.[8]

He argues that benefit estimates are expensive, not only in terms of the dollars and staff resources required, but also because they delay the implementation of regulations aimed at correcting serious problems and divert an agency's resources from other serious issues. The increased uncertainty is inherent in the estimation process, for each step of the analysis has to build upon and therefore incorporate the uncertainty of the previous step. There are also methodological problems that tend to increase the uncertainty of more elaborate estimates: the inherent uncertainty associated with making any projections, controversy in some instances about what are benefits and what are costs, and the question of the appropriate discount rate to use when comparing future costs and benefits with current costs and benefits.

Benefit analyses may decrease the amount of *useful* information provided by obscuring relevant information and by either ignoring or forcing quantification of essentially unquantifiable factors. One particularly thorny problem, on which there is no agreement, is the precise value to place on a human life. Also, highly quantified estimates ignore information on the distributional impacts—the issue of who benefits and who pays for past or proposed actions. This is quite important, since the basic issue with most health regulation is who benefits and who pays. Do the workers and nearby residents pay

by being exposed to unhealthy conditions, while the firm and its customers benefit from lower prices, or vice versa?

The bias problem involves not only the hidden, often substantial, biases of the practitioner, but also several ways in which the methodology of benefit-cost analysis is itself biased. In addition to its blindness to distributional considerations and its likely treatment of the future as being less important than the present, a third methodological problem is that benefit analyses are normally based upon averages because the average is considered to be the best single representation of a distribution. The importance of the often substantial deviations from the average is thereby hidden. A final methodological problem, which aggravates many of those mentioned, is that economic analyses implicitly assume that all situations are reversible. Yet, irreversible decisions may have very high costs, and therefore such actions should perhaps be avoided. However, there has been very little thought about how to deal with such problems: there is now no way to deal with them quantitatively, and they are rarely addressed in quantified benefit analyses.

Robert Haveman compiled an excellent summary list of the problems to date regarding studies of the economic benefits from air and water pollution control. He reached the following conclusions regarding air pollution, the focus of this section:

1. The theoretical basis for estimates of the health effects of residuals concentrations is very weak. For most of the important relationships, the relevant epidemiological data is unavailable. In addition, as Lave has noted, there are numerous unanswered questions of a conceptual, empirical, and statistical sort. Most fundamental is the difficulty of separating the health effects of pollution from health phenomena that are influenced by a large number of other, nonpollution-related and pollution-interrelated variables. Analogous problems afflict estimates of soiling and materials damage effects from air pollution.

2. In the absence of specified general equilibrium models, the effect of air pollution levels on property values cannot be known. The meaning of the "willingness to bid" functions that have been estimated is not clear. They appear to have been overinterpreted, given the absence of such general equilibrium models.

3. The studies on soiling, materials damage, and vegetation effects of air pollution have been weak in the specification of the concept of damages and its relationships to the standard welfare economics framework. This, in addition to the lack of data and the absence of knowledge of physical effects, makes these studies of little use.

4. Studies that seek to estimate damages by asking people what they would pay to avoid various levels of residuals concentration or noise

are likely to be of little use. Two problems appear fatal. First, there is substantial reason to believe that respondents' perception of damage and increased risks is sorely inadequate. Second, because of the public goods nature of the pollution problem, interviewees have incentive to understate their willingness to pay if it is anticipated that the costs of damage reduction will be related to their statements.

5. While most of the air pollution damage studies have yielded estimates of national damages, most of the important public decisions must be local or regional decisions. They include the setting of emissions standards for various kinds of pollutants and sources, setting of relevant emissions charges, the establishment of zoning regulations, or the undertaking of abatement investments. Such national estimates are of little help for these decisions. While such estimates could possibly be of help for, say, national decisions on research investments in transport systems as alternatives to automobiles, they are too unreliable to offer much assistance.[9]

The final report of a joint EPA—Penn State University project to evaluate current environmental research and establish priorities focused in its economic solutions section on ways to improve benefits analysis. Specifically, the economics committee recommended five ways to improve EPA's ability to determine the economic benefits of its pollution control activities:

1. By developing a detailed methodology for defining and measuring health status sufficiently sensitive to low levels of encroachment on individual functioning and relevant to behaviorial analysis.

2. By investigating the relative effects of environmental factors on health status while controlling for differences in lifestyles, genetic makeup, economic status, demographic factors, and the availability of health services.

3. By analyzing people's use of the natural environment as a function of the quality of the environment.

4. By analyzing avoidance activities and other behaviors intended to offset negative environmental effects.

5. By analyzing the economic valuation placed on physical decrements in the environment in relation to other values and opportunities.[10]

ENVIRONMENTAL PROGRESS IN THE 1970s The most obvious and direct benefit from environmental protection measures is the improvement in pollution levels that has taken place. A report released in 1979 cited the following improvements for the period 1972 to 1977:[11]

- Sulfur dioxide levels dropped 17 percent
- Carbon monoxide levels were cut 20 percent
- Particulates (smoke and dust) decreased 8 percent, resulting in an estimated 18 million fewer people being exposed to levels violating health standards in 1977 than in 1972
- Ozone levels showed little change despite a 30 percent increase in motor vehicle miles traveled

There has also been significant progress in the area of water pollution. Our rivers and waterways are much better off now than they were in 1970. Many that were literally "dead" or contained little aquatic life are on their way back to normal.

A GENERALLY POSITIVE IMPACT ON ECONOMIC ACTIVITY

An increasingly critical question in recent years has concerned the impact of environmental regulations on the performance of such key economic variables as growth, employment, prices, and productivity. The general impression conveyed by the mass media is that the barrage of "nonproductive" expenditures has had a highly negative effect and has been a primary contributor to the nation's recent economic woes.

Actually, such a perspective is quite distorted. When the full evidence is examined and environmental expenditures are viewed in the necessary comprehensive perspective, they are seen to have had some direct positive impacts as well as having helped to rectify a fundamental failure of the market pricing system.

GNP Growth and Employment

The fundamental (yet often forgotten) point about environmental expenditures is that their impact on macroeconomic activity heavily depends on the general state of the economy. In a tight economy, such expenditures will likely increase prices and replace other capital spending plans with a relatively small employment effect. However, in a slack period, such as that which characterized much of the 1970s, pollution control expenditures can stimulate growth and employment with little real effect on prices.

Econometric analysis has confirmed this positive impact. A Data Resources, Inc. study released in January 1979 estimated that the GNP at that time was slightly higher than it would have been otherwise due to federal pollution requirements causing capital and other resources to be used that would not have been used under the slack economic conditions of the 1970s.[12]

Employment in the 1970s also benefited. DRI estimated the 1979 unemployment rate to be 0.2 percent lower due to federal pollution

requirements. This is not to say that no negative employment effects occurred. EPA's Early Warning System identified nearly 25,000 job dislocations between 1971 and June 1979 where pollution control costs were alleged by companies to be a significant factor. Nevertheless, this is only an average of 3,000 jobs per year in a labor force which averaged over 90 million over the same period. Environmental regulations can also reduce employment when the price increases that accompany pollution control requirements result in decreases in demand.

These negative impacts are more than offset by the many ways in which employment is stimulated by environmental requirements. Jobs are created directly through the construction of wastewater treatment facilities. It is estimated that each billion dollars for such construction produces 15,000 work-years onsite and 19,500 offsite ($24.5 billion has been authorized by Congress for the next five years).[13] Currently, nearly 36,000 people are employed in the pollution control manufacturing industry, with growth to 44,000 projected by 1983.[14] In addition, there are hundreds of thousands of workers employed in industry whose primary responsibility is pollution control, either in the design, construction, operation, and maintenance of pollution control equipment, or in the development of process changes to comply with requirements.

As for the 1980s, the DRI model estimated that GNP will be about 1.0 percent lower in 1986 than it would have been without federal pollution requirements. Employment, on the other hand, will be positively stimulated—the unemployment rate is projected to be 0.4 percent lower in both 1980 and 1981 and 0.2 percent lower in 1986 due to federal pollution control requirements.

Prices and Productivity The positive impacts on growth and employment are virtually neglected in the popular press, which focuses on the added inflationary pressures and productivity inhibiting effects of environmental requirements. Though there is a measure of truth in each of these charges, it is a very incomplete measure, which thereby distorts the real impact.

The incomplete measure regarding prices takes the form of the DRI estimate that the CPI in 1979 was about 2.7 percent higher than it would have been without federal pollution requirements and that by 1986 this difference will be about 3.6 percent. This translates into a rather small 0.2 to 0.3 annual percentage point increase in the CPI in the period to 1986, but any increase is seen as a "call to arms" by some critics.

One fundamental problem is that such estimates of the impact of environmental spending on the CPI show price increases resulting from pollution control costs, but they do not reflect the savings accruing to consumers in the form of reduced medical costs, reduced

time off work due to illness, improved recreational opportunities, increased crop yields, and reduced property damages (not to mention the immeasurable benefits of reductions in pain or discomfort). It the value of these additional outputs from environmental regulations is more than the increased costs, the regulations are not truly inflationary.

There are three major weaknesses of the CPI as an indicator of real inflation:

- It does not take account of shifts in the patterns of consumption.
- It does not take adequate account of changes in the quality, as opposed to the price, of goods.
- It does not include a number of nonmarket goods that are important to the overall quality of life.

The first of these problems concerns the fact that pollution control programs result in reduced consumption of such items as medical services and surface coatings. Such defensive expenditures do not really add to the quality of life but only help prevent it from becoming worse. The second problem is that price increases that reflect the true cost of pollution control should not really be treated as price increases at all. A prime example of where this has been recognized and taken into account is new car prices. The Department of Labor, arguing that new cars are actually better cars because they emit fewer pollutants, attempts to adjust for this "quality" improvement by deducting the cost of pollution control devices from new car prices before these are entered into the CPI calculation. The same holds true for increased monthly electric bills, which represent an increase in value in the product itself—cleaner electricity costs more than dirty electricity. A reasonable quality adjustment for goods in general, if the benefits of the reduced emissions exceed the associated abatement costs, would be to deduct the embodied pollution abatement costs from the price of the product before determining whether its real cost had increased. If such adjustments were made for all products, pollution control programs *could not* be inflationary. The necessity of making these types of quality adjustments is the third problem area cited above.

Due to these many problems, we have no true measure of the impact of environmental regulations on prices—one that takes into account both the increased prices and improvements in the quality of life.

We also forget that the relative rise in prices as a result of pollution controls is simply a means of putting the market mechanism to work to protect the public health and welfare. It is, thus, not clear conceptually why greater costs and uncertainty should discourage investment as long as firms can raise prices to cover the higher costs and obtain compensation for their greater risk. The higher prices are likely to

dampen demand, but this is desirable to the extent that it results from consumers bearing the full costs, including the environmental costs, of producing the product. By allowing industries in the past to use environmental resources at no cost, we have encouraged them to expand at the expense of those resources. An increase in relative prices, which both discourages the purchase of environmentally intensive goods and encourages the development of less-polluting industrial processes, must be a central part of an efficient environmental protection program.

Thus, far from being interferences in the free market system, the Clean Air Act and the Water Pollution Control Act were necessary corrections where markets had failed. Whether these corrections were excessive depends on a careful accounting of costs and benefits. In theory, however, they are perfectly consistent with, and indeed called for by, a properly functioning, free market economy.

There has also been much recent concern over the impact of environmental regulations on productivity. Most of it stems from a 1977 study by Edward Denison in which he attempted to quantify the reduction in annual productivity increases due to the diversion of business capital and labor to environmental control.[15] He found that by 1975 the imposition of environmental controls made output per unit of input in the nonresidential business sector of the economy 1.0 percent lower than it would have been if business operated under 1967 conditions. The study carried with it the mystical aura of a highly quantitative approach, and most of the mass media accepted it as the final word.

Like all quantitative estimates at the present state of the art, this study suffers from a number of limitations. First, Denison's methodology identified all incremental business expenditures on pollution control as diversion from investment that would have produced measured output, rather than attempting to take into account the data indicating that over one-fifth of pollution control investment is for change-of-process rather than add-on technology. The two forms of compliance have quite different effects on productivity gains. A related, and most important limitation, is his invalid assumption that every dollar spent on pollution control results in a dollar less of so-called "productive" spending. Individual companies do not make dollar-for-dollar substitutions of this type, because they will frequently raise additional money that allows profitable investment in some "productive" investments that would have had to have been dropped if only a fixed amount of capital were available. The models of Chase Econometrics and Data Resources, Inc. use an investment reduction coefficient of 0.3 to 0.4, which means that a $1.00 expenditure for pollution control equipment leads to a $.30 to $.40 reduction in other capital expenditures.

Denison also did not attempt to take into account the decrease for some industries in pollution damages over the 1967 base, which are due to other industries' environmental control effects. Finally, he limits the study to productivity rather than attempting to assess the efficiency of the regulations by comparing benefits with the productivity losses.

Thus, Denison's study is far from a serious indictment of environmental regulations. It is a useful additional input into the slowly evolving process of more accurately assessing the quantitative impacts of environmental regulations on economic activity.

In thinking about the impact of environmental regulations on growth and productivity, we would do well to adopt Paul Samuelson's perspective. After referring to his Net Economic Welfare construct, which tries to take into account the improved amenities that "are just as important to each living generation as the mousetraps and the other ordinary things," he concludes:

> When you have calculated these auxiliary measures of physical production and of corrected Gross National Product then it's not the case that investment in pollution control equipment is nonproductive and is a subtraction from what could otherwise have been produced. On the contrary, it may be that in any one year's spending on these items in a society not at the bare margin of existence these may be among the most important welfare-creating expenditures.[16]

STIMULUS TO INDUSTRIAL INNOVATION

One of the principal benefits of environmental regulations—which has virtually gone unrecognized and certainly has not been included in any quantitative impact analyses—is that they have been the most important single force in the post-World War II era in terms of causing American industry to rethink and change established production and management processes on a wide scale. Though most firms have not yet responded by implementing process changes, a significant number of firms have reexamined their production processes in evaluating compliance alternatives and made minor modifications. A smaller number of firms (but a continually growing number) have reevaluated their entire production system and have developed superior processes or process controls, which not only solved pollution problems but directly led to the adoption of more economic processes or processes that saved energy.

A two and one-half year study at the Massachusetts Institute of Technology confirmed that regulations have had a positive impact on innovation.[17] The regulation/innovation relationship was analyzed in five industries (auto, chemical, computer, consumer electronics, and textile) in five countries (France, Germany, Holland, the United

Kingdom, and Japan). The study found that innovations for ordinary business purposes were much more likely to be commercially successful when environmental/safety regulations were present as an element in the planning process than when they were absent. In addition, compliance-related technological changes often led to product improvements far beyond the scope of the compliance effort. The study also concluded that many direct attempts of governments to encourage innovation were not correlated with project success to as great an extent as was regulation.

The following chapter develops this benefit theme in much greater detail.

FOOTNOTES TO CHAPTER 3

1. Lester B. Lave and Eugene Seskin, "Air Pollution and Human Health," *Science,* 1970, pp. 723–733.

2. Lester B. Lave and Eugene Seskin, *Air Pollution and Human Health,* Johns Hopkins University Press, 1977.

3. Ronald G. Ridker and John A. Henning, "The Determinants of Residential Property Values with Special Reference to Air Pollution," *Review of Economics and Statistics,* May 1967, pp. 246–257.

4. Thomas Q. Crocker, "Urban Air Pollution Damage Functions," presented at the Econometric Society meetings, New Orleans, December 1971.

5. Crocker et al., *Methods Development for Assessing Air Pollution Control Benefits,* Volume 5, Executive Summary, Environmental Protection Agency, February 1979.

6. Ibid., p. 15.

7. Ibid., p. 21.

8. Edwin H. Clark II, "Arguments Against Undertaking Formal Quantified Benefit Estimates for Health and Environmental Regulations," internal EPA paper, Novermber 1, 1978.

9. Robert H. Haveman, "On Estimating Environmental Damage: A Survey of Recent Research in the United States."

10. *Cooperative Agreement for the Evaluation of Current Environmental Research and Establishment of Priorities,* Pennsylvania State University, Program in Health Planning Administration, October 1, 1979.

11. *National Air Quality, Monitoring and Emissions Trends Report, 1977.*

12. Data Resources Inc., "The Macroeconomic Impact of Federal Pollution Control Programs, 1978 Assessment," Boston, January 11, 1979.

13. Fact Sheet, *EPA Journal,* January 1979, p. 15.

14. Arthur D. Little, Inc., *The Economic Effects of Environmental Regulations on the Pollution Control Industry,* Cambridge, Mass., September 1978.

15. Edward Denison, "Effects of Selected Changes in the Institutional and Human Environment Upon Output per Unit of Input, *Survey of Current Business,* January 1978.

16. Paul Samuelson, "An Economist's View," *EPA Journal,* January 1979, p. 5.

17. Center for Policy Alternatives, MIT, *National Support for Science and Technology: An Examination of Foreign Experience,* CPA Document 75-12.

4

ENVIRONMENTAL REGULATION AND TECHNOLOGICAL INNOVATION

TECHNOLOGICAL INNOVATION IN THE UNITED STATES TODAY

Speaking woefully of the decline of American technology has become fashionable. Some observers attribute this downward trend to the web of regulations that allegedly limits companies' resources and strangles their incentives to innovate. This chapter disputes that theory and discusses what government can do in the 1980s to ensure that regulations not only have a minimal inhibiting effect but also work increasingly toward stimulating innovation.

A General Assessment

Those who argue that the United States is in technological decline are able to marshal an impressive array of supporting evidence and statistics, mostly related to research and development (R&D) expenditures. As a percent of the GNP, R&D spending peaked in the middle 1960s and declined until 1978. R&D spending for basic and exploratory research, measured in price adjusted dollars, has been on a plateau for ten years. Because private spending for R&D from 1970 to 1977 was lackluster, its percent of the GNP was lower in the United States than in Germany or Japan.

Such statistics are part of a broader and more fundamental phenomenon, which Jerome Wiesner, while he was president of MIT, referred to as "technological maturity." The argument—that much of the innovative thrust of corporations seems to have dissipated as several vital postwar industries have reached a mature stage—has also been sounded by business leaders. Jacob Goldman, group vice-president of Xerox Corporation, believes there has been a decline in innovation and a shift toward simply improving the old; while Jerry Wasserman, a senior consultant with Arthur D. Little, contends that most so-called innovations build on existing technologies and simply extend the state of the art. Jay Forrester, an MIT professor who was instrumental in computer development in the 1950s, is forcefully succinct: "Our present technology is mature. Since 1960 there has not been a major radically new, commercially successful technological innovation comparable to aircraft, television, nylon, computers, or solid-state electronics."[1]

Historically, theory maintains that as an industry matures, it becomes more resistant to new technology. The financial and organizational commitments to old ways of doing things are simply too great to make major changes. This argument has been used to explain why there were virtually no important technological advances in automobiles after the introduction of the automatic transmission in the 1930s until the new electronics of the mid-1970s, and why Europe and Japan have surpassed America in steel technology.

Statistics from *Science Indicators 1976* bear out the "building on existing technologies" theme. From 1953 to 1973, the fraction of major innovations that could be called "radical breakthroughs" declined from 36 percent in 1953-59 to 16 percent in 1967-72.

Although the overall assessment is generally somber, there are some bright spots. Industry's total R&D expenditures increased 16 percent in 1977 and 10 percent in 1978, reaching $21.8 billion. Most significantly, in recent years corporate laboratories have been turning out a stream of major developments, primarily in the electronics field but also in energy and biology.

Indeed, in sharp contrast to the maturity of basic industries, industries in the electronics, communications, and information field are bringing about what is increasingly referred to as an information revolution. While much of industrial technology was relatively crude, requiring only a modest scientific or theoretical base, the information revolution is the product of the most advanced scientific knowledge, technology, and management and represents a great intellectual achievement.

In the search for new sources of energy, the federal government and more than 100 companies jointly funded (at a total cost in 1978 of $2.7 billion) a number of projects to convert coal into cleaner burning or more easily transportable fuels, such as high-octane gasoline. Recently, scientists have made major breakthroughs in nuclear fusion by using lasers, rather than magnetic forces, to focus the enormous energy needed to fuse hydrogen atoms and create a nuclear reaction. Other scientists believe the most promising energy research may lie in the large-scale production of hydrogen as a replacement for gasoline, natural gas, and other fuels.

Genetics and microbiology are also fertile fields for innovation. There is general agreement that microbiotics research has far-reaching commercial potential. Gene splicing may eventually be used to create new varieties of crops, as well as new strains of bacteria, for such purposes as converting garbage to methane gas or concentrating valuable metals from low-grade ore.

In addition to these corporate lab developments, industry is making some of its most important technological gains in the soft technology of systems engineering. Systems engineers, the generalists of industrial

research, create technologies by merging developments from unrelated fields in ways that might not be apparent to specialists. Outstanding examples are the space program and Bell Laboratories' pioneering work in glass fiber cables.

Government's Effect On Innovation: Mixed Review

Governments in all developed countries work to promote and shape technological development because it is the most important contributor to a nation's economic growth. A 1977 Commerce Department study found that from 1929 to 1969, technological advances were responsible for 45 percent of America's economic growth.[2] It also revealed that from 1957 to 1973, technology-intensive industries' output, employment, and output per worker grew 45 percent, 83 percent, and 38 percent, respectively, faster than that of other industries; prices, however, increased only half as fast.

Yet, the private market has many inherent limitations in coordinating all the effects of technological change. For example, it can do little to control such adverse effects of technological change as unemployment, pollution, and unsafe products. Since private firms also cannot capture all of the benefits arising from innovation, they will tend to underinvest from a societal viewpoint. Moreover, the limited scale of most firms prohibits their undertaking large-scale or risky developments. In other cases, the public interest will require a government role in shaping new technological development that private firms may not pursue (for example, pollution control research or transportation facilities for the handicapped and elderly).

Many, if not most, government programs were not originally intended primarily to affect innovation, but embraced a wide variety of independent societal goals. For the most part, policy toward innovation remains only implicit in many political decisions. Although no major, across-the-board support for basic civilian technology exists, there are three key forms of intervention: research, procurement, and regulations.

There is little disagreement about the positive effect of the first two forms. Outstanding contributions to industrial innovations from government basic research include its work on aerodynamics, high-temperature liquid cooling, and improved aviation fuel. Government procurement also has great strategic leverage in stimulating innovations in product areas with commercial growth potential, a prime example being establishing aircraft designers as commercial innovators.

The effect of regulation on technological innovation, however, is a highly debated topic. Discussion of this issue is often clouded by emotions raised by the larger issue of the desirability of regulation. Thus, considerable care must be taken, through a comparison of costs and

benefits, to separate the treatment of the effects of regulation on technology from the societal value of regulation.

Popular writings generally inveigh against the stultifying effects of regulation—particularly the relatively recent barrage of environmental, health, and safety (EHS) regulations—on innovation. Actually, very little empirical evidence on the subject exists, and the few studies that do attempt to measure these effects reach conflicting conclusions.

Perhaps the most definite conclusion that can be drawn is that general, sweeping conclusions concerning the effects of regulation on technological change must be avoided. Regulation seems to have both hindered and stimulated innovation. Much depends on the timing and quality of a regulatory intervention. If the needed infrastructure, which includes trained people is not in place or is created concurrently to meet the regulatory requirement, severe dislocations may result. Also, intense pressure for rapid change may force industry to patch up an existing technology rather than risk the failure of a radical innovation. On the other hand, when regulation is steady and gradual and firms have sufficient time to comply, effective and innovative technological solutions often appear.

We can also conclude that because EHS regulation affects the industrial process at different states of product development and production, it will have a variety of effects both on its stated goals of improved health, safety, and environmental quality and on technological innovation. For instance, regulations requiring companies to demonstrate product safety or the efficacy of products before marketing may produce effects different from those requiring such safety or control after marketing. And the effects of regulations requiring the control of production (process) technology, or effluent emission or waste control, or the safe transportation of hazardous material will also vary.

EFFECTS OF ENVIRONMENTAL REGULATIONS ON INNOVATION The complexity of the regulation-innovation relationship precludes the possibility of deriving a final number that summarizes the net impact. Part of the complexity lies in the distinction that must be drawn between the direct effects on innovation in compliance efforts and the longer-term, ancillary effects on the general process of business innovation. Either effect is likely to vary significantly, depending on the nature of the regulation and the regulated industry.

As shown below, environmental regulation has stimulated and retarded both forms of innovation. Since such effects cannot be summed, it is impossible to assert that the regulation has exerted an overall net change in the rate of innovation. What is clear, however, is that the innovation process has been redirected toward new social

purposes.

The degree to which firms positively respond to calls for innovation depends largely on the incentives built into the environmental laws and regulations. The United States has given insufficient attention to using regulatory legislation to encourage the production of compliance technologies to achieve regulatory goals. Certainly, the regulations themselves do not effectively stimulate such new technologies or production processes. This contrasts sharply with the experience of several other countries, where approaches to regulatory design often focus specifically on new technology. Following is a critique of those provisions in the laws and regulations that relate in some manner to innovation.

Law and Regulations Are Not Innovation Oriented   Although a few provisions of the Clean Air and the Clean Water Acts provide incentives for new corporate pollution control strategies, they have stimulated few innovative compliance responses. Once polluting industries are in compliance, they have very little incentive to seek improved environmental performance.

The provisions most directly related to innovation are the innovation waiver permits of the 1977 Clean Air Act amendments. With regard to existing sources, Section 113(d)[4] states that the EPA Administrator can waive the requirements of state implementation plans (SIPs) for up to five years if the polluting source:

1. Proposes a new means of emission limitation
2. Can adequately demonstrate this new technology by the end of the period
3. Promises that the new technology will result in either:
   a. better performance
   b. lower cost
   c. lower non-air environmental impact
4. Can not install and test the new technology without the waiver

Section 111(j) outlines a similar program for new sources. The proposed system:

1. Must receive a public hearing
2. Must have the state government's approval
3. Must not have been proved
4. Must have "substantial likelihood" that it will achieve either:
   a. better performance
   b. lower cost
   c. lower non-air environmental impact

The waiver cannot run longer than seven years from issuance and four years after the new source starts operation.

The primary benefit of these provisions could be to allow the long-term operation of pilot or large-scale test facilities. However, since the Acts require compliance at the end of a period that is much too short to allow significant depreciation of capital, these provisions do not provide any real incentive to build a commercial facility that has potential benefits but risks not achieving performance standards. Reflecting this problem and the lack of publicity on these provisions is the fact that as of November 1979, only one application out of 23 had been granted a waiver.

Congress viewed the new source performance standards in the 1977 amendments as "technology forcing" provisions that would stimulate innovation and environmentally improved production processes. The requirement that new sources achieve performance corresponding to the best demonstrated technology was originally intended to provide the incentive of an assured market to developers and vendors of improved controls. The incentive has proven to be remarkably weak.

The phrase "technology forcing" describes a regulatory provision that goes beyond a voluntary incentive to bring forth new technology. The CAA amendments use it in three contexts: nonattainment regions, nondeterioration regions, and state petitions. The "technology forcing" provision (Section 173) requires new sources locating in nonattainment areas to use "lowest achievable" emission rates. Section 165 applies a "best available" criterion to control technology for any emission source in a nondeterioration area. After Congress modified the bill, the distinction between "best available" and "lowest achievable" was essentially nonexistent. Finally, Section 111(g)[4] allows a state to petition EPA to upgrade new source standards, with the availability of technology as an acceptable rationale.

A final innovation-related provision of the CAA amendments is the offset policy for nonattainment areas. It deals with the key question of how to initiate a process that will stimulate industrial innovation designed to improve environmental as well as economic performance.

The offset policy is one of a number of economic incentives in effect or under consideration by EPA. Bill Drayton, while EPA's Assistant Administrator for Planning and Management, emphasized that offsets and other economic incentives such as the bubble policy, reinforced by the banking of reductions and the use of deal-making brokers, are critical for increasing the rate of innovation in control technology. In a study of economic incentives, two of the three advantages cited were that they create a better climate for technological change, directly encouraging it in some cases, and they encourage innovation.[3]

The 1977 Clean Water Act (CWA) amendments demonstrate the determination of Congress to advance the use of innovative and alter- 63

native technologies in sewage treatment. The amendments state that in providing grants or subsidies, EPA will prefer those systems that "incorporate wastewater reclamation and energy recovery, as opposed to the conventional concept of treatment by means of biological or physical chemical unit processes and discharges into surface waters."

The amendments contain three interlocking financial preferences, in the form of direct capital subsidies rather than tax subsidies, for communities that invest in new technology for reutilizing sewage in publicly owned waste treatment plants (POWT). The major one, Section 202(a)(2), increases the federal cost share from 75 percent of a POWT's construction cost to 85 percent if a community uses an innovative approach. This provision is a strong incentive because it represents a 40 percent capital cost reduction for the localities.[4] A further inducement is the lower relative operating costs of nondischarge approaches— costs that localities generally have to pay in full. Under Section 202(j), an innovative grant application may show estimated life-cycle costs of up to 15 percent more than the conventional guidelines technology and still be approved. Finally, Section 202(a)(3) provides that if an innovative or alternative technology project fails, the government may give the community a 100 percent grant to fund its modification or replacement costs.

The CWA amendments relate to innovation in three other ways: they require that innovative and alternative technologies be studied and evaluated for all projects, they provide a 15 percent credit for cost-effectiveness analysis in evaluating such projects, and they allow states to modify their priority lists to give greater preference to such projects.

Although the Toxic Substances Control Act does not have any innovation-specific provisions, Section 2(b)(3) contains perhaps the clearest legislative expression of the importance of technological innovation to those involved with both industrial production and improving worker and consumer safety or the environment.

> It is the policy of the United States that. . . authority over chemical substances and mixtures should be exercised in such a manner as not to impede unduly or create unnecessary economic barriers to *technological innovation* while fulfilling the primary purpose of this Act to assure that such innovation and commerce in such chemical substances and mixtures do not present an *unreasonable risk* of injury to health or the environment." [Emphasis added.]

The Act does contain a provision allowing companies to share testing costs for particular chemical products that may be an important benefit to small firms' innovation efforts. Broadly viewed, TOSCA could improve the climate for innovation in the chemical industry by replacing much of the present uncertainty with preestablished and

well-defined procedures.

Besides enacting the environmental laws, Congress has enacted a number of tax incentives for pollution control. On the whole, these tend to bias corporate decisions toward end-of-pipe conventional control technologies rather than innovative, preventive process changes.

The Revenue Code contains two major tax benefits that reduce the cost to firms of complying with pollution control regulations: (1) rapid amortization and the investment tax credit for pollution control hardware, and (2) tax exemptions for municipal bond financing of pollution abatement facilities.

The Code's accelerated depreciation provision (Section 169) allows pollution control hardware to be amortized faster than other equipment. Although the deduction applies to both pollution abatement and prevention, the nonsignificant change requirements severely restrict the latter—namely, preventive facilities *cannot* lead to a significant increase in output, capacity, or the useful lives of equipment; a significant reduction in operating costs; or a significant alteration in the nature of the manufacturing process or facility. "Significant" is defined to be more than a 5 percent change. A related provision allows the investment tax credit to be claimed for one-half of the costs qualifying under Section 169.

Often, firms do not use these provisions because they find that using only the full investment tax credit is more beneficial. When they are used, they tend to bias environmental compliance. Since companies can clearly identify only end-of-pipe technologies as pollution control investments (because they find it difficult to identify operations and maintenance expenditures that are included in process change control efforts as an investment per se), they tend to adopt those techniques that are easily subsidized (and thus made artificially less expensive) rather than more efficient change-of-process controls. Furthermore, the nonsignificant change requirement provides substantial bias toward incremental or patch-on, rather than major, process changes.

Two studies for the Office of Technology Assessment and the National Bureau of Standards support these conclusions:

> . . . the current tax treatment for pollution-control expenditures appears to have simply encouraged retrofits on existing facilities instead of investment in newer and more efficient technologies.[5]

> . . . the liberal tax treatment for investment in general appears likely to work against innovation in the short-run, having a greater relative impact on the expected return to conventional technology.[6]

Finally, EPA influences the utilization of control technologies through its research and development and its technical assistance. In the past,

R&D concentrated on end-of-pipe control technologies that may have contributed to the underrepresentation of process change. Recently, the focus has shifted to process change, but it is too early to assess the impact. In the past, EPA's technical assistance efforts have also favored end-of-pipe controls. Since process changes are more case specific than end-of-pipe controls, EPA engineers asked by industry to provide technical assistance often recommend controls based on their general applicability.

Environmental *Compliance* *Innovation* Although it is clear that regulations encourage technological change in compliance responses, such changes will not necessarily be "innovative." Indeed, the question of whether the technology-based approach has encouraged innovation is still subject to much controversy.

Critics of the approach have argued that perverse incentives for technological innovation are inherent in the way technological requirements are framed. Company officials, for instance, may reason that if they do not meet the effluent limitations, they will be safe from EPA prosecution as long as they have made a "good faith" effort to achieve the standards by adopting the suggested strategy. If this is true, the technology-based approach may encourage a risk-averting strategy of adopting the suggested or sanctioned technologies, even when they may be expected not to meet the standards. Also, in cases where the regulatory standard is set at the level of the best practice in a few leading firms, the major effect is diffusion of an existing technology to the lagging firms rather than innovation.

On the positive side, it can be argued that by requiring dischargers to control their emissions to levels that engineers say can be achieved, a technology-based policy forces the adoption of the best available technology (BAT). Other counterarguments suggest that: (1) sufficiently strong commercial incentives exist to produce high-standard equipment; (2) there is evidence that applying suggested technologies does not hinder innovation; (3) no firm is permanently exempt from BAT regulations; and (4) a noncompliance fee can be levied.

A study by the Organization for Economic Corporation and Development (OECD) summarizes the situation well:

> ...although technology-influenced effluent standards may appear to be determinent and objective, in practice, many controversial judgments and decisions appear to have been made in translating the legislative directive to base effluent limitations on technological considerations into specific numerical limitations. ...The technology approach is *not* neat and simple compared to the messy complex value judgements that are associated with ambient environmental standards, setting effluent charges and so forth.[7]

Ancillary Innovation   As for the longer-term, ancillary effects on the general process of innovation, the accumulating evidence suggests that environmental regulations provide a very healthy stimulus that is likely to outweigh any negative effects.

Looking first at the negative aspects, regulation can diminish conventional innovation by reducing the overall R&D budget, by diverting R&D funds from conventional to compliance research, and by changing the allocation of funds in conventional R&D activities. Although these effects are widely perceived to be significant, evidence on the magnitude of these effects does not exist. Furthermore, only a small fraction of the money spent on industrial R&D is going into pollution control R&D—3 percent in 1977.

Another alleged negative impact is that environmental regulations accelerate the technical and economic obsolescence of equipment, since the old equipment not only is generally more polluting but also necessitates larger expenditures to make it conform to the new standards. Although this effect does exist, it is not necessarily negative, since the regulations simply accelerate inevitable trends.

On the other hand, an MIT study confirmed that regulations can have a positive impact on innovation.[8] The study analyzed the regulation/innovation relationship in five industries (auto, chemical, computer, consumer electronics, and textile) in five countries (France, Germany, Holland, the United Kingdom, and Japan). It found that innovations for ordinary business purposes were much more likely to be commercially successful when environmental/safety regulations were present as an element in the planning process than when they were absent. In addition, compliance-related technological changes often led to product improvements far beyond the scope of the compliance effort. The study also concluded that many direct attempts by governments to encourage innovation were not correlated with project success to as great an extent as when regulation was used. Another study, by the Science Policy Research Unit of the University of Sussex, suggested that environmental regulation in the six countries studied did not appear to have prevented or delayed innovation to a significant extent and may even have had a "substantial stimulating influence on improving quality and performance."[9] Finally, the OECD reports that environmental regulation has (1) helped Japan develop cheap alternatives to PCBs and devise new techniques to meet strict auto emission standards, (2) stimulated the development in Norway of a cheaper energy-saving alternative to open-furnace burning, and (3) stimulated an effort in France to recover many unrecovered pollutants for their economic value.

Looking more specifically at the United States, there is an often overlooked but very significant stimulus to general business innova-

tion—process change, which often yields economic or energy-related benefits. The thesis is that environmental regulation often shocks firms out of a rather inflexible production system, thereby providing the catalyst for innovation to occur. A number of studies provide evidence supporting this thesis. The Denver Research Institute found "strong support" for the idea that the need to change occasioned by regulation provides an opportunity to make process improvements in areas unrelated to regulation.[10] A study of the effect of environmental regulations on the industrial chemical industry reported that 33 percent of its respondents cited indirect benefits relative to process improvements.[11] Another study of this industry found that the people interviewed thought the new analytical capability needed to assess the health/environmental risks of both new and existing products would be important for the future development of products and processes.[12]

It should also be recognized that the emergence of a new sector—the pollution control industry—shows governmentally stimulated innovation on a large scale. The industry's performance in 1972-76 reveals better than average growth but only average profitability. In 1977, the markets for pollution control products totaled $1.8 billion. These markets are projected to grow to $3.5 billion by 1983, a pace of 11-12 percent per year. Furthermore, the industry and the technologies it uses show a very favorable balance of payments, with the United States maintaining a position of great strength in world markets.

Regulation-Induced Process Change

While it may be concluded that most firms have not responded to regulation by implementing process changes, it is also true that environmental regulations have been the most important single force in the post-World War II era in terms of causing American industry to rethink and change established production and management processes on a wide scale. Moreover, while a large majority of firms have responded to the Clean Air and Water Acts' requirements by applying end-of-pipe controls (either out of necessity or unwillingness to engage in more creative thinking), a small but significant number of firms have evaluated compliance alternatives and have often made minor modifications in their production processes. In a growing number of cases, firms have thoroughly reevaluated their entire production system and have developed superior processes or process controls that not only solved pollution problems but led directly to the adoption of energy-saving or more economic processes. Based on a 1977 survey of industry, the Census Bureau estimated the value of the energy and materials recovered as a result of pollution control measures to be more than $950 million.

Most of the process changes are specific to a given company, but the
auto industry's use of electronic microprocessors to control engine

performance for both fuel economy and lower emissions levels provides a striking example of an industry-wide change. Philip Caldwell, vice chairman and president of Ford Motor Company, actually refers to the "opportunities" provided by government regulation that have initiated "revolutionary change" in auto design and that are creating a "great new market."[13] He maintains that typical cars of the 1980s will be 100 percent more fuel-efficient than those of 1974, resulting from an "explosion" of new applications in electronics and other "explosions in materials substitution and the use of computer technology in design and manufacture."

The auto industry's adoption of microprocessors illustrates three important principles. First, regulation can create the impetus for transferring technology from one industry to another. For example, a large market has been created for firms producing such devices as microprocessors and sensors. Second, new technologies sometimes provide great potential for expanding and improving their application, in this case for other electronic automotive applications such as controlled braking. The third, perhaps most important, principle, is that actions that complement the normal competitive pressures for change on an industry often appear to be more effective in promoting innovation than those that do not relate to market forces. Industry thus finds itself doubly motivated to innovate.

Following are examples of companies that have reevaluated their production processes, leading to the adoption of innovations that resulted in significant economic and/or energy benefits:

Economic and Energy Savings

■ *Glass Containers Corporation* has developed the largest glass recycling program in the United States and has made technological discoveries that will increase recycling nationwide. By using a much higher percentage of used glass in a batch of molten glass and developing a computerized control system for using waste glass in the batch, the company reports that air quality improvement has been so great that no special pollution control devices have been necessary for furnaces, and that fuel savings and longer furnace life have resulted. This system provides an additional economic benefit to cities and towns faced with expensive landfill problems.

■ *Uniroyal Chemical,* to better dispose of hundreds of thousands of gallons of nonenes (a form of chemical waste), devised a process to combine the nonenes with fuel oil and burn them in the company's steam-generating boilers. During the first year of operation, the process recovered and burned 366,000 gallons of waste nonenes, resulting in substantial fuel oil savings. Against investment costs of $48,000, first-year savings from the changeover were about $183,000.

■ *Long Island Lighting Company* used a magnesium fuel additive to 69

reduce sulfur trioxide concentrations. Burning magnesium oxide with its Venezuelan fuel oil not only solved the environmental problem but also produced a marketable by-product, vanadium. In 1978, the company sold 362 tons of recovered vanadium for $1.2 million, and saved $2 million in fuel because of thermal efficiencies and $400,000 because of reduced boiler corrosion.

Economic Savings

■ *Gould, Inc.*, began replacing more traditional wastewater treatment methods with a reverse osmosis cleansing process that permits its plants to recycle most of the water they use. Savings from the system—which allows recovery of large quantities of copper, conservation of sulfuric acid used in plating, and achievement of several other economies—are expected to exceed $450,000 a year, thus recovering the $845,000 system installation costs in less than two years.

■ *Great Lakes Paper Company* installed an $8 million closed-cycle water treatment system, which is expected to save $4 million each year in lower costs for chemicals, water, and energy, while containing contaminated effluents.

■ *Hercules Power* spent $750,000 to reduce solids discharged into the Mississippi River. As early as 1971, it was saving $250,000 a year in material and water costs.

■ Process improvements in a *Gold Kist* poultry plant cut water use by 32 percent, reduced wastes by 66 percent, and produced a net annual saving of $2.33 for every dollar expended.

■ *Centron Corporation* developed a system to recover solvent vapors which were previously expelled into the atmosphere, from the production of magnetic tape. Estimated savings are $50,000 a year, but actual savings are much higher since the firm can now use less expensive, nonexempt solvents in the process. (Air pollution from solvents has dropped from 450 tons to 59 tons per year.)

■ *J. R. Simplot* virtually ended its discharge altogether with a system combining primary treatment of its liquid effluents and spray irrigation. The system has eliminated from nearby streams and groundwater almost all of the 40,000 pounds of biological oxygen demand, the nutrients, and the suspended solids. Moreover, the plant now sprays the nutrients in the wastewater on the land to produce high protein forage, which it combines with other solid wastes from the plant to feed 26,000 yearling steers. The waste heat in the effluent used to irrigate the land allows a 10- and 11-month growing season and an annual yield nearly twice that of normal croplands in the area.

■ *Dow Corning* found that a $2.7 million capital investment in equipment to recover chlorine and hydrogen previously lost to the atmosphere reduced operating costs by $900,000 a year—a 33 percent annual return on investment.

Energy Savings   ■ *The Aluminum Company of America*
developed a way to recycle fluoride in its
refining and smelting process and thereby eliminated the need for huge
quantities of water. In addition to significantly reducing fluoride fume
emissions, Alcoa's new fluidized bed technology cuts energy
consumption in two processes by 30 percent.

■ *Corning Glass Works* devised an improved, electrically powered
melting process that eliminated the loss of certain raw materials to the
air. The process has vastly reduced air emissions and simultaneously
allowed better control over glass production. Energy consumption has
been reduced by a factor of 3.7 in the new plants, and the reduced space
required for building this system has lowered construction costs.

■ *The Georgia-Pacific Corporation* developed a special scrubbing
system to eliminate "blue haze" emissions caused by plywood production. Collecting the airborne pitch produced a thick liquid, which has a
Btu rating that is the equivalent of #6 fuel oil. The firm now uses this
residue as a fuel supplement, and the four units in operation collect
enough residue to replace 51,000 gallons of #6 fuel oil each year.

■ *The Florida Power Corporation* installed burners that were designed to operate at very low levels of excess air. This development
simultaneously increased boiler efficiency and lower fuel consumption. It also reduced visible emissions from 40 percent to 10 percent
(state standard is 20 percent). After one year, Florida Power's ten
burners have consumed 4,000 fewer barrels of oil than with the previous system. And the new system reduces operating costs because it
requires less manpower.

■ *Wheelabrator-Frye* found that converting garbage and refuse to
energy could be a practical enterprise. The firm constructed a facility
on a former landfill site. The facility receives all of the garbage from
Boston's thickly settled North Shore and processes it, producing eco-
nomical steam energy for a nearby General Electric plant. This system
has made cheaper steam energy available and has reduced refuse disposal costs to the North Shore communities. In addition, it saves 27
million gallons of fuel oil a year.

The fundamental principle that all of these examples illustrate so well
is the strong link between management commitment to compliance
and the nature of the effect of regulation. Strong management
commitment normally results in both lower compliance costs and
favorable effects on innovation.

One company that has had such commitment and results is the 3M
Company. In 1975, it introduced the Pollution Prevention Pays (3P)
program to stress conservation-oriented technology that will prevent
pollution at the source in products and manufacturing processes rather
than remove pollution after it is created. This is a continuing effort that   *71*

focuses on eliminating pollution sources through product reformulation, process modification, equipment redesign, and the recovery of waste materials for reuse.

As of 1979, 39 projects selected for recognition had annually eliminated the equivalent of 75,000 tons of air and 1,325 tons of water pollutants, 500 million gallons of polluted wastewater, and 2,900 tons of sludge. In three years, the total estimated saving was about $17.4 million, mostly from eliminated, reduced, or delayed capital pollution control investment and operating costs, including savings from improved products and processes, and some sales retained from products purged of a pollutant or toxic compound. Ten overseas subsidiaries had their own programs, which undertook 75 projects, representing an additional savings of $3.5 million.

An example of a 3P project involved recycling cooling water that had previously been collected for disposal with wastewater. Reusing the cooling water allowed the capacity of a planned wastewater treatment facility to be scaled down from 2,100 to 1,000 gallons per minute. The recycling facility cost $480,000, but 3M saved $800,000 alone on the construction cost of the wastewater treatment plant.

After three year's experience, the company was pleased with the results and remained as firmly committed to the program as it was when it started. According to Joseph Ling, vice-president for environmental engineering and pollution control:

> Necessity, the cliché goes, is the mother of invention. This may be an overworked phrase, but that makes it no less true—particularly in reference to pollution abatement. 3M's attention was directed toward pollution control initially because of necessity. Now it is directed toward elimination of pollution sources for the same valid reason—it is necessary. The cost of relying entirely on pollution removal technology—the little black box at the end of the pipe—simply is becoming too great, considering the myriad other demands on our financial resources.[14]

This is precisely the type of resource-conserving philosophy leading to action that must become widespread throughout corporate America in the 1980s.

SHAPING AN INNOVATION/INDUCTION PROGRAM

Encouraging Resource-Conserving Technology

In the 1980s, there will be a new approach to pollution abatement—developing resource-conserving technology that will both conserve resources and lower the cost of pollution abatement by working to eliminate the sources of pollution in processes and products before waste is created. If waste is broadly viewed as the "irrational use of more than necessary

resources to fulfill human needs and objectives," resource conservation becomes "a positive image for the application of technology to fulfill human needs and aspirations without destructive impact on the environment."[15]

Over the long run, this type of technology will be much more environmentally effective and cost-efficient than the traditional end-of-pipe control measures so heavily relied on in the 1970s. The main problem with the latter "removal" technology is that it only contains the problem temporarily. Such measures that are subservient to the immutable Law of Conservation—we can change the form of matter but it will not disappear—do not solve the problem but merely shift it from one form of pollution to another.

Removal technology presents a number of other problems. Control measures create "off-site" pollution, which is pollution generated by those who supply the materials and energy consumed in the pollution-removal process itself. Also, the cost of pollution control, the resources consumed, and the residue produced increase exponentially as removal percentages rise to the last few points. At this stage, eliminating the final stage of pollution often can create problems many times greater than those that were eliminated.

Thus, using only the control approach to solve environmental problems is contrary to the objective of a resource-conserving society, which should instead change pollution-abatement philosophy and adopt resource conservation-oriented abatement technology. This change—a simple concept, but with profound implications—is no more, and no less, than the practical application of knowledge, methods, and means to provide the most rational use of resources to improve the environment.

Resource conservation technology means eliminating the causes of pollution before spending money and resources to clean up afterward, as well as learning to create valuable resources from pollution. In short, the concept is to use a minimum of resources and create a minimum of pollution.

There are at least four major environmental and economic benefits of an approach that increasingly substitutes pollution-source elimination for pollution-control technology:

■   It allows us to save energy and other valuable resources that can be applied to other problems and can provide opportunities for human betterment.
■   Since little, or in certain instances, no waste is generated, pollution problems are eliminated once and for all.
■   The new technological spin-offs could offer innovative opportunities to convert waste materials considered as pollution today into valuable resources for other constructive uses tomorrow.

■ It is the most effective, long-range solution to the increasingly serious and complex global environmental problems.

A resource-conservation approach also helps eliminate a type of pollution left untouched by the control approach: the environmental impact of products after they leave the factory. Since a product is likely to contain any number of pollutants, a problem is created for the user that is beyond solving by controls in the manufacturer's factory. If the user is another manufacturer, the "within the product" pollution could become a "within the manufacturing process" pollution problem. The vicious circle can only be broken by eliminating the pollutant from the product in the first place through resource-conserving technology. For example, by removing a mercury catalyst from an electrical insulating resin, the 3M Company did away with any pollution problem the mercury created for the user. The new formula was more environmentally acceptable and helped 3M prevent a substantial loss in sales.

Resource-conservation technology is neither a panacea nor a substitute for pollution control. Some industries cannot easily change their processes without disrupting or halting production. Changeover may be too costly, or there may be no resource conservation technology to eliminate the pollution sources.

The goal should be to use resource conservation technology where and when it is possible and practical. Individual industries must apply their ingenuity to develop their own techniques relating to their special pollution problems. Over the long run, the resource-conservation approach should prove to be more environmentally effective and less costly than conventional control methods.

Implementing Legislative and Regulatory Reform To encourage the development of both the new technologies necessary to achieve environmental goals and safer products and materials, Congress should resolve to increasingly consider issues concerning regulatory system design and implemention. The debate concerning environmental regulation, focusing on the need for new legislation and the *stringency* of regulatory requirements, has underemphasized questions relating to implementing the legislative mandates. Various ways of promoting the growth of innovative compliance technologies include government support for efforts to achieve regulatory goals through technological change, effluent taxes, and provision for joint research and development for pollution control.

Perhaps the most direct and effective action can be taken in drafting regulations. In the 1980s, there should be two corresponding policy goals vis-à-vis innovation toward which environmental regulations should work:[16]

■ To the extent that they are consistent with the environmental-safety goals established by legislation, regulations should not unduly hamper innovation for ordinary business purposes.

■ To the extent possible, regulations should encourage innovation in compliance and abatement technology. This innovation should both address alleviating the immediate hazard and contribute to longer-term systemic changes that can result in more environmentally benign and safer products and processes in the future.

The goal is to design regulations that will advance both goals. Where these two goals are inherently incompatible, however, difficult policy trade-offs will have to be made between them.

One of industry's most frequent complaints is that the compliance period specified in regulations is too short to allow for development of the most effective or innovative response. For example, the 3M Company states that "legislation and regulations usually provide neither the time nor the flexibility a company needs to develop products and processes which eliminate or reduce pollution at the source; the rules are directed primarily toward achieving pollution removal."[17]

The validity of this type of complaint is open to some question in that a several-year period of government scrutiny, hearings, and public controversy precedes most regulations. During this period, industry receives a clear signal of the standard to come. Nevertheless, it is true that developing important compliance innovations (especially those involving relatively major changes in existing technology) can take a number of years. In such cases, extending the time period between standard promulgation and full compliance (i.e., timing) could serve as a means of encouraging innovation. A closely related idea is to more effectively use the experimental waiver provisions in the Clean Air and Water Acts. High-risk but strong candidates for advancing state-of-the-art technology should be more easily granted waivers in situations with low exposure and low adverse environmental hazard potential. Possible abuses can be controlled by specifying a limit on the number of waivers per industrial category or control type.

The experience of Glass Containers Corporation provides an example of the benefits that can accrue from flexibility in extending a compliance deadline. EPA first gave the company until June 1976 to comply with air quality standards. But when the company did not meet that deadline because it was having trouble finding enough used glass for its new recycling process, the EPA regional office granted it a six-month extension. Company officials enthusiastically responded to this flexibility:

> They could have come in here at any time and just said "do it now," and
> we might have cut our operation in half. Instead, they were patient,

worked with us...now we are working full shifts around the clock, paying out well over $1 million to the local economy, keeping thousands of tons of glass out of the solid waste landfills, and turning out bottles as good as they have ever been.[18]

Much could be done in R&D to promote innovative responses and resource-conserving technology. Regarding federal R&D generally, any significant federal program designed to foster the development of new technologies should be required to evaluate the comparative environmental and economic advantages of the proposed technology. Regarding environmental R&D, the federal effort should be expanded to include work on improved generic methods for waste reduction, separation, and disposal. In addition, some industries sorely lack research and innovation on systematic approaches to simultaneous process and pollution control design to minimize overall production costs. Such approaches need to be developed for industrial processes, integrated manufacturing plants, and area-wide waste management.

Another broad government-wide reform concerns the contract and grant specifications of federal agencies. All federal agencies—particularly those like DOD, GSA, HUD, and DOT—that purchase directly or control the purchase of manufactured goods can provide a major incentive for industry to use processes that pollute less and to develop products with the least possible environmental impact. This objective could be furthered by inserting clauses in the contract and grant specifications that favor government or government-subsidized purchases of the most environmentally safe products or of products derived from the most environmentally benign processes.

Another possible regulatory reform is to replace the substance-by-substance approach with a "generic" standard for a class of substances. The generic approach greatly reduces regulatory uncertainty. Because it gives firms a clear and advance signal of the kinds of substances that will likely be regulated and the nature of the controls that will probably be required, it allows the private sector to develop appropriate, long-term technological options.

EPA should explore the merits of a privately administered revolving fund to partly ensure against developmental cost losses when products are not registered (pesticides) or cannot be produced due to general regulatory provisions (chemicals). This would help alleviate the problem of companies that tend to hold back on developing new products because of their perception of the difficulty of getting new products registered or approved and the financial loss involved if their registration application or premarket notification is rejected.

A report to the Congressional Office of Technology Assessment offered a list of regulatory alternatives that may foster innovation:

1. Expansion of direct government support for in-firm technological development in crucial areas (e.g., pollution control in automobiles) leading to both process and product change.

2. Modification of pollution control tax incentives, i.e., accelerated depreciation and municipal bond financing, so as to favor process redesign and the development of new products and materials rather than add-on modifications associated with purchasing of pollution abatement equipment.

3. Government financial support for major new technological advances when firms are unlikely to undertake them on their own, either because such development would require large-scale efforts, would be long in coming to fruition, or would have nonappropriable results (e.g., closed systems to contain toxic chemicals). This occurs in Germany and France as part of broader programs to encourage the development of new technologies for various social purposes.

4. Greater industry-specificity in standard setting (e.g., in the OSHA context) so as to minimize hardship when new technologies would be difficult to develop, and to maximize health safety protection when the technological capacity is great.

5. Alternative or supplements to standard setting such as products liability or strict liability imposed on polluters, as in Japan.

6. A formal antitrust exemption procedure to clarify the status of joint R&D relating to environmental control technology.

7. Special programs to assist small firms' compliance efforts.

8. Effluent taxes as a means of achieving water pollution abatement on a regional basis (these have apparently been successful in Europe, especially in Germany, and are alleged to provide continuing incentives for more efficient control technology).[19]

What this list and the preceding suggestions primarily illustrate is the need for a thorough reassessment of the means of achieving regulatory goals via technological innovation. Such a reassessment must begin now if the United States is to become a resource-conserving society in the 1980s.

FOOTNOTES TO CHAPTER 4

1. Jay Forrester, "Changing Economic Patterns," *Technology Review,* August-September, 1978, pp. 52-3.

2. Cited in "Vanishing Innovation" *Business Week,* July 3, 1978, p. 47.

3. James Booth and Zena Cook, "An Exploration of Regulatory Incentives for Innovation: Six Case Studies," Washington, D.C.: Public Interest Economics Center, January 18, 1979.

4. It should be noted that since wastewater treatment funding has been without ICR systems for much of the grant program, firms have been subsidized for the dumping of their wastes. Thus, the 75 percent subsidy likely has led ultimately to a disproportionte use of end-of-pipe controls.

5. Center for Policy Alternatives, MIT, *Government Involvement in the Innovation Process,* Washington, D.C.: Government Printing Office.

6. Booth and Cook, op. cit.

7. OECD, *The Influence of Technology in Determining Emission and Effluent Standards,* Paris, 1979.

8. Center for Policy Alternatives, MIT, *National Support for Science and Technology: An Examination of Foreign Experience,* CPA Document 75–12.

9. Science Policy Research Unit, University of Sussex, *The Current International Economic Climate and Policies for Technical Innovation,* November 1977, p. 20ff.

10. Boucher et. al., *Federal Incentives for Innovation,* Denver Research Institute, University of Denver, January 1976.

11. J.C. Iverstine, *The Impact of Environmental Protection Regulations on Research and Development in the Industrial Chemical Industry,* National Science Foundation, May 1978.

12. Center for Policy Alternatives, MIT, *Environmental/Safety Regulation and Technological Change in the U.S. Chemical Industry,* 1979.

13. "Caldwell Lauds Regulation as a Spur to Innovation," *Automotive News,* January 22, 1979.

14. Joseph T. Ling, "Pollution Prevention Pays," *Pollution Engineering,* May 1977, p. 33.

15. These definitions are from a seminar sponsored by the U.N. Commission for Europe on "Principles and Creation of Non-Waste Technology and Production."

16. These two principles were put forth by Ashford et. al., in *The Implications of Health, Safety and Environmental Regulations for Technological Change,* Center for Policy Alternatives, MIT, January 15, 1979, pp. 3–2 & 3.

17. Ling, op. cit., p. 34.

18. Larry Kramer, "Bottle Maker Cuts Costs, Pollution with Old Glass, *Washington Post,* July 2, 1978.

19. Center for Policy Alternatives, MIT, *Government Involvement in the Innovation Process,* op. cit., 59–60.

5

ENVIRONMENTAL QUALITY
AND ECONOMIC GROWTH

**THE BASIS OF
THE PARTNERSHIP**
The expression "everything is connected to everything else" is commonplace and universally accepted. Yet, only in recent years have economists and environmental scientists come to recognize the influence each one's field has on the other. Even then, the influence has been viewed only as a negative one—with environmental scientists thinking that economic growth inevitably brings environmental harm and economists thinking that environmental regulations, of necessity, adversely affect economic performance. Indeed, in the past year or two, it has become fashionable to assail environmental regulations as a major contributor to increased prices and decreased productivity and, hence, the country's economic woes.

This mutual neglect and suspicion are ironic in light of the fact that the words "economics" and "ecology" share the same root, "eco"— derived from the Greek word for a house or home. Ecology can be viewed as the study of the natural mechanisms of resource dynamics (or nature's housekeeping), and economics as the human process of managing resources (or human housekeeping).

From this perspective, there is no excuse for neglect. It has been clearly documented that economic factors have been in the past (and will be in the future) one of the predominant determinants of environmental needs and demand as well as of environmental policies themselves. It is equally clear that environmental phenomena have pervasive global and regional consequences that not only alter the conditions and the quality of human life but also may affect and endanger the process of economic production.

The adversarial relationship that has developed is as ill founded as the neglect of the one for the other. This is not to say that economic activity has not harmed the environment or that environmental regulations have not adversely affected economic activity. The distortion of the truth lies in the exclusive focus on such effects, neglecting the important nuances and the way in which economic and environmental principles and policies are, or can be made to be, compatible.

For example, the weight of the evidence indicates that is is less the fact of growth than the manner of growth and the uses made of it that lie at the bottom of environmental problems. The thrust of the

productive technologies developed and employed since World War II have constituted a counterecological pattern of growth.

The time has come to explicitly recognize that growth need not in and of itself cause pollution, nor environmental protection measures limit growth. Indeed, the United States must continue to vigorously pursue its environmental goals while enjoying the best of its economic and physical growth.

The critical questions are: What patterns of growth are anticipated in the 1980s? And what can be done to shape a pro-ecological pattern of growth? The pattern will be determined chiefly by the transformation in the economic structure from one based primarily on manufacturing and industry to one based primarily on information, knowledge, and communications. Since the "information revolution," as it is increasingly referred to, is extremely sparing of energy and materials, it will help foster greater environmental quality in the 1980s by producing much less pollution in the first place.

Such change, while helpful, is not sufficient. In the 1980s, we will have to operate with explicit societal goals as the quality of economic growth. Setting such goals could be facilitated through in-depth analysis of the relationship between rates and patterns of economic growth and various degrees of pollution control to help determine which combinations are capable of meeting environmental standards. For example, eight scenarios could be examined: high and low resource-intensive economic growth with high and moderate pollution control, and high and low resource-conserving economic growth with high and moderate pollution control. After determining which combinations would meet environmental standards, alternative economic/technological/environmental policies could be explored to determine the most desirable growth pattern.

In the 1980s, we must move beyond the trade-off mentality—economic growth vs. (or) environmental quality—and recognize that the two are not only mutually compatible but complementary in many ways. Alfred Kahn, former President Carter's anti-inflation chief, emphasized this complementarity:

> Environmental values *are* economic values; it is in principle just as important, in the interest of economic efficiency and therefore economic welfare, to conserve our limited natural resources, to make wise and sparing use of our limited clean air, water, and living space, as it is to economize in the use of labor and capital; and using some of our limited economic resources to preserve or restore an acceptable environment is just as much a contribution to economic welfare as devoting them to travel, shelter, or national defense.[1]

80 Much depends on the types of technologies adopted. Increasingly,

major technologies to be introduced must be treated as dependent variables that can and must be channeled in accordance with our environmental objectives. Most broadly, we must compare alternative interventions in the system in terms of their overall effects on environmental quality and economic performance. Such analysis would likely uncover a wide range of options that might improve both the economy and environmental conditions, thus demonstrating the complementarity referred to above.

Beyond such analysis, we must continue to develop and more effectively use economic incentives in environmental policy-making as well as integrate physical principles into economics and economic policies.

ECONOMIC INCENTIVES IN ENVIRONMENTAL REGULATIONS

Throughout the 1970s, environmental protection was pursued largely through the setting of standards, a "command and control" approach that entailed deadlines and a considerable degree of government scrutiny. Standards are, however, only one of many possible mechanisms that might be used to achieve environmental goals. Economists have long advocated the use of economic incentives as an attractive alternative or supplement to the existing approach.

In the past few years, EPA has examined several forms of economic incentives. These reforms seek to avoid the conflict between environmental objectives and the demand for industrial growth, as well as meet increasing complaints that environmental regulations are starting to provide less pollution reduction at greater cost. The set of interdependent reforms, known as "controlled trading," includes offsets and the associated banking and brokerage concepts, the bubble policy, and marketable permits. All look toward development of a market in air pollution emission reductions, overseen by state and local air pollution control agencies through existing permitting processes. The approaches differ from each other only in terms of how the "commodity" to be used in trading is defined and initially located, the rules of the market, and whether trades occur within a single industrial facility or between different plants.

The offset policy has been in effect since 1976, while the bubble policy was implemented in December 1979. The approaches are closely related, both allowing increased pollution to be balanced by compensating decreases of the same pollutant from other sources. Because business firms have considerable freedom to choose the polluting operation from which to reduce emissions, these approaches can accomplish pollution reduction at the lowest possible cost.

The use of marketable permits as a way of first allocating and then letting permit holders transfer to others some or all of their rights to

emit pollution was studied for EPA by the RAND Corporation. The study focused on permits to emit fluorocarbons, but the concept clearly has broader potential application.

After examining EPA's two operational policies—offsets and the bubble policy—this section will examine the theory and applicability of emission charges and conclude with a general assessment of economic incentives.

The Emissions Offset Market

"If from any revolution in nature the atmosphere became too scanty for the consumption...air might acquire a very high marketable value." A little over a century after John Stuart Mill wrote those words in 1862, air officially acquired a marketable value in EPA's Interpretive Ruling of December 21, 1976. Henceforth, nonattainment areas could permit industrial growth from major new construction or major modifications of existing polluting sources only if the new source provided for an offsetting reduction of emissions within the area. Why and how did such a market for air pollution get established?

In the mid-1970s, it became apparent that progress toward meeting national air quality standards was too slow, and thus EPA grew less inclined to grant emergency variances and other types of exceptions to its regulatory deadlines. Simultaneously, it was recognized that the air quality standards allowed little room for industrial growth in regions that were behind schedule in achieving cleaner air. For example, a major new emission source (one emitting more than 100 tons of certain pollutants annually) was not allowed in a nonattainment area. Thus, the pressures for industrial development and employment and income growth hit the inflexibility of EPA's national standards head-on. It appeared that, within a short time, industrial expansion would come to a halt.

In the last half of 1976, certain kinds of internal trade-offs were allowed on a case-by-case basis. Plant-specific emission entitlements had begun to emerge, and property entitlements in air quality use had reached the barter stage. Though not intended as such, a crude and limited market was taking shape. Due to considerable public interest in the trade-off policy, EPA sought public comment on the idea through its December 1976 interpretive ruling. The 1977 amendments to the Clean Air Act allowed this ruling to continue in operation for nonattainment areas until July 1, 1979. After July 1, 1979, the states were given a choice of two options for handling new growth: create a quantitative margin for growth with the State Implementation Plans (SIP) by imposing emission limitations on existing sources to a greater degree than minimally necessary to meet standards or continue some form of case-by-case emission offset approach. Any nonattainment

area not covered by a SIP that ensures regional achievement of national air quality standards by December 31, 1982, will face a ban on new major sources of emissions.

The problem the offset policy addresses is not a small one. There are hundreds of nonattainment areas that exceed one or more of the six ambient air quality standards EPA enforces. In mid-1978, Los Angeles violated five standards, while four were violated by such major cities as Philadelphia, Chicago, Cleveland, and St. Louis. Without the offset policy, economic growth in these areas would be severely retarded.

The "rules of the market" are quite simple.

1. Offsets may be created in a number of ways, including (a) a decree of a governmental body (i.e., a demand that existing sources reduce pollution), (b) cooperation among firms (e.g., Chambers of Commerce may encourage existing firms to surrender offset credits), or (c) the purchase of offsets from existing sources.

2. In treating its discharge, new major emission sources must use a technology that yields "the lowest achievable rate of emission" (LAER). This means that a new source cannot gain additional emission entitlements by shifting from an inferior to superior technology. Nor can it sell existing entitlements if new, cleaner technology is developed.

3. Only the same kinds of emissions are subject to exchange. For example, only emissions of sulfur dioxide may be substituted for emissions of sulfur dioxide.

4. An emission offset of more than one-for-one is required, or, to put it another way, each transaction carries an in-kind tax.

5. Only parties desiring to build new emission sources can enter the market as buyers. Proponents of improved air quality cannot buy emission entitlements and destroy or hold them.

6. All existing facilities in the state owned by the new or modified source must be in compliance with the State Implementation Plan (SIP) or on an approved compliance schedule.

7. The offsetting emissions must be calculated from the level of the applicable SIP (A source out of compliance must measure offsets from the SIP rather than from the actual level of emissions).

To the buyer of the emission offset, it is an additional expense that must be incurred in order to construct a polluting facility. The emission offset is not a permanent "privilege or entitlement to pollute." The future environmental, technological, economic, and regulatory framework that the source will be subject to is unknown. Therefore, the cost of the offset can be treated as a one-time start-up cost. To the seller of the offsets, an offset is simply compensation for an unrequired reduction in its emissions.

In designing an offset policy appropriate to particular nonattainment areas, an efficient emission control program recognizes that control can most easily be implemented on those types of sources that simply require recently demonstrated technology. Area-wide planning could take advantage of potential trades from these sources and provide incentives through an offset policy to reach the standard. A large industrial or utility firm needing an offset (in order to build a new plant) would be encouraged to organize and finance the introduction of a technology to control some other major source of emissions in the area.

There are many advantages of the offset market. Perhaps the principal one is that it promotes economic efficiency, allowing firms with potentially high emission control costs to gain exemptions by facilitating the attainment of other lower-cost firms. Emission entitlements are allocated to those firms producing the greatest economic benefits to society. Each firm can assess its particular environmental situation and seek the lowest cost solution. For example, firms are prompted to consider the relative merits of different locations, production processes, and emission-control systems as well as the relative merits of controlling additional emissions or allowing them to go uncontrolled by incurring the cost of permits or fees. In economist's jargon, the opportunity cost of the environment is made explicit.

The other major advantage is that paying for air emission entitlements makes the value of air quality clear to both buyers and sellers, thus leading to conservation and efficient use of pollution control devices. Moreover, the fact that emission entitlements have a cost is likely to cause firms to search for alternative methods of producing their products, thus creating an additional incentive for discovering and implementing new control technologies. This is quite important, for the current system provides disincentives for the development of new technologies to the owners and management of pollution sources. Further control of those sources must be brought about primarily by providing the owners and managers economic incentives to develop more advanced control technologies.

An extremely important feature in helping the offset market run smoothly is the newly developing area of "banking" of emission reductions. This should encourage firms to anticipate the demand for offsets by controlling emissions more than the law requires. Since firms with lower control costs will be able to sell their offset for less and are more likely to attract customers, they will have a considerable incentive to find the most effective, efficient control systems. To encourage the activities of brokers needed to facilitate trades, EPA is working to set up information clearing houses so that firms seeking offsets can easily locate firms wanting to sell them.

Banking of emission entitlements is potentially an important instrument for shaping local development. If emission entitlements can be purchased for future use from a firm closing a plant or otherwise willing to reduce emissions, a local or state development agency could purchase them as they become available. It could either sell the emission entitlements or use them in a manner similar to tax abatements as industrial location incentives. The emission entitlements could be used to ensure that firms with high jobs (or income) to emissions ratios are induced to locate in the area.

The offset market has two other advantages. First, as compared with an emissions charge scheme, it reduces administrative costs by relieving administrators of the need to set a charge for pollution entitlements and to change that charge periodically to reflect regional economic growth and decline. Second, it separates the property right (entitlement) to environmental use from the discharger's other assets, thereby making the property right fully transferable, a feature that satisfies the preference for contractual solutions.

Despite these important advantages, the offset market is far from being a perfect solution. Two possible problems, common to any marketable permits-like system, could emerge in a less-than-ideal competitive market—problems that would make it at least questionable whether the determined price could be presumed to accurately reflect the utility to society of using the environment as a sink for dispersing and absorbing pollutants. One problem is that powerful corporations might use pollution entitlements as a means toward monopoly by refusing to sell them to existing or potential competitors. The second problem is that collusion might occur among cooperative bidders with a common interest in minimizing the cost of such entitlements. Given the results of auctioning off other public goods such as offshore drilling rights, it is far from clear that the market will operate in a pure and straightforward manner.

In alleviating the problem of constant adjustment of fees, the offset market creates the problem of freezing any overly optimistic decision made about the level of pollution that a given environment could be expected to absorb. Any later decision to raise the quality of air through decreasing the number of pollution entitlements on the market faces the seemingly insurmountable obstacle of clearly defined property rights and their traditional protector, the judicial system. If, on the other hand, the level of property entitlements in pollution were set so low as to produce an unrealistically clean environment, there would be—in addition to the obvious possibility that officials responsible for distributing and policing them could be corrupted—continuous pressure from the community at large to expand a too-limited supply. It is likely that the factors influencing decision-makers to expand those entitlements would increase in direct proportion to the

increase in density of industry and population. Also, whenever the economy entered a slump, additional pressures would arise to "find" or to create new pollution entitlements to sell.

Emission entitlements, like any property right, require government protection. If it is uncertain that government will protect emission entitlements, firms will sharply discount their future value, and only those transactions that give promise of high return will be likely to occur. EPA officials could reduce uncertainty and thereby push forward the investment horizons of emission entitlements purchasers by carefully defining all emission entitlements and by strictly enforcing requirements that emissions be monitored. State authorities could add protection to the new property entitlements by keeping other air quality users from "poaching" and by ensuring some minimum life to them at the time of an approved exchange.

In addition to the problems created by changes over time, there is the problem of distributing the costs of cleanup equitably. In order to achieve maximum utility of the assimilative capacity of the environment, it is necessary to sell pollution entitlements at varying locations. Thus, dischargers could become increasingly concerned about inequities in assessing entitlements as finer and finer distinctions were drawn among different locations in the same general region. Zones, however drawn, must have boundary lines; dischargers located on different sides of those lines would inevitably make comparisons.

The more than one-for-one offset is a further problem. Although it leads to reduced emissions when trade-off transactions are made, it is also likely to reduce the number of transactions that occur since it makes emission entitlements more expensive when traded than when held (that is, there is a tax on the transaction). This will encourage less-efficient users of these entitlements to hold on to—and use—those they have, rather than trading them to more efficient users. The efficiency of the market is thus substantially reduced.

Perhaps the fundamental problem boils down to the unsettled question: What is the optimal amount of air quality to be marketed? Without a definitive answer to this question, total efficiency will not be achieved through the offset market.

The Bubble Concept
In January 1979, EPA proposed the bubble concept to allow sources greater flexibility in efficiently controlling their air emissions. The flexibility is created by placing an imaginary "bubble" over all or part of a plant. The owners of plants can meet their emission reduction requirements by putting extra controls on discharge points within the plant with lower control costs, in exchange for easing the pollution control requirements for discharge points with high control costs. Trade must be made between discharges of the same pollutant.

Consider a simplified example: a single plant with two boilers, each of which is limited by current regulations to emitting no more than 50 tons of pollutants a year. One boiler burns high-sulfur coal and is producing 60 tons a year; the other is burning low-sulfur oil and is putting out 40 tons a year. To comply with existing regulations, the plant is forced to burn a mixture of both fuels in each boiler. That means building a pipeline from the oil burner to the coal burner and renovating each boiler to burn the fuel of the other. Under the bubble concept, the limit would be 100 tons for the two boilers together. No investment would be needed, and the overall air quality would be the same.

As originally proposed, the policy only applied to Prevention of Significant Deterioration (PSD) or "clean" areas, not nonattainment or "dirty" areas. The final policy announced in December 1979 allowed the bubble's use in nonattainment areas that had demonstrated to EPA's satisfaction that they would attain standards as of a certain date. A D.C. Circuit Court opinion on the bubble policy expressly disallowed its use in regard to New Source Performance Standards.

The bubble policy's effect on industrial innovation is a matter of dispute. Some argue that it encourages plant engineers to find the most cost-effective mix of pollution controls to meet the standard and thus provides an incentive for industrial innovation. Others argue that since a company must meet the schedule of existing regulations—even if the company is drafting an alternative plan under the bubble concept—engineers do not have sufficient time for innovative thinking.

Another alleged problem is that it is virtually impossible to prove in advance that any substitution of one emission for another is an "even" trade, unless the two pollutants are absolutely identical. The fear is that EPA will, therefore, create not one or two bubbles over a plant, but many small bubbles—one over stacks, one over storage piles, one over roads, and so on. To the extent this occurs, the system will simply imitate old-fashioned stack-by-stack regulation.

The concept has the potential of achieving a sensible balance between environmental controls and costs and stimulating industrial innovation. Still in its early stages, it is too early to judge whether it will achieve these goals. Only if and when industry begins to come forward with innovative proposals will it become clear whether state officials have enough flexibility to permit creative economizing.

Emission Charges

The approach most favored by economists, and hence most prevalent in the literature on economic incentives, is the emission (or effluent) charge (also referred to as tax or fee).[2] Economists find the underlying logic simple and compelling. If the damage caused by different concentrations of residuals were known, the environmental regulators would simply

establish a charge or price equal to the marginal damage for each unit of residuals. Polluters would decrease their residuals flows as long as the marginal cost of doing so was less than the price for discharging, settling at the opitimum where marginal treatment costs equaled the charge.

Economists cite a number of major advantages. Perhaps the most important is that it would allow individual waste dischargers, who are presumably best informed about the relevant technologies, considerable discretion in the method they choose to deal with their wastes. It is assumed that residuals' managers would thereby arrive individually at the most economically efficient solution for their own units and collectively for the society as a whole. Total control costs would be lower than under most regulatory programs because there would be more control by polluters with low abatement cost, and less by those with high abatement costs.

With respect to economic efficiency and environmental effectiveness, emission charges are the converse of standards. Given a set of ambient standards and appropriate enforcement procedures, emission standards can always be calculated so as to satisfy the environmental objective, but there is no way of knowing whether the objective will be met in an economically efficient manner. On the other hand, for any given level of emission charges, the resulting reduction in pollution is achieved at the least cost, but there is no guarantee that the charges will be sufficient to meet the environmental standards.

In addition to increased efficiency in the use of societal resources, economists argue that effluent charges would promote greater administrative effectiveness than possible under the standards approach because so much responsibility has been transferred to the polluters. Polluters are forced immediately to make decisions that save them money based on the full cost to society of their actions. Since the the charges are presumably imposed without qualification, tendencies to procrastinate, to seek legal relief, and to resist research expenditures are lessened. When action is necessary, enforcement officials who have been hesitant in using court cases, injunctions, and large fines would be likely to enforce emission charges more strictly. Instead of a complex bureaucratic process in which multiple opportunities exist for negotiation between regulator and regulated, there would be a simple fee schedule requiring fewer administrative decisions and allowing for less discretion in enforcement. In general, by incorporating the economic value of the environmental resource directly into the polluters' decisions, a charge system would eliminate the need for regulatory agencies to calculate an optimal level of controls for society.

It is also argued that charges are equitable in the sense that every polluter would have to pay society the real cost of using scarce environmental resources, and none would be faced with marginal

control costs that are much more or much less than the cost to society of pollution damages.

Why, given such advantages, have emission charges not been used by EPA? First, the advantages are not really as clear-cut as they seem, and there are a host of serious real-life implementation problems, which the theory tends to gloss over. Even the foundational allocative efficiency advantage has been subject to serious questioning recently.

It has been noted that is the tax does not capture all of the costs of pollution *and* if firms do not recognize the hidden costs of pollution to themselves, the firms' decision to either pollute or pay the tax will be a less correct one and an insufficient amount of compliance will occur. While raising the level of the tax can increase compliance in the aggregate, allocative efficiency may not be as great as one might expect if the hidden costs of pollution to the firm are large and vary significantly from firm to firm. A number of firms will continue to make suboptimal decisions between compliance and paying a tax, unless a tax is set on a company-specific basis, which is unlikely to occur.

It has also been pointed out that as the discharge control target is raised, the costs of treatment associated with the tax will rise relative to the standards approach. At high levels of control, as in the Clean Air and Water Acts, the "efficiency advantage" of the tax approach declines sharply from the advantages that show up at lesser levels of controls.

Some economists have gone so far as to demonstrate that, under certain circumstances, allocation of specified wasteload reductions to each discharger (as in the present system of permits and standards) can produce *more* efficient results than a uniform charge for each type of waste. This occurs whenever the marginal cost for treatment by individual dischargers is sufficiently varied to produce different responses from each when a uniform fee is applied, but when environmental conditions are such as to demand equal treatment from all. Physical variables related to both time (e.g., seasonal flow of water) and space (e.g., inversion-prone airsheds) may affect environmental quality to the point where uniform emission charges prove as unresponsive to actual needs as do uniform reduction standards.

The most basic problem with implementing emission charges is that insufficient data currently exist to set an emissions charge equal to the damages to society for each polluter's wastes. Without this information, it is impossible to use emission charges to ensure an optimal level of pollution control for society. To the extent that control costs or current emission levels are not known, a charge system would be less certain than a standards approach in reaching precisely the desired level of control. Thus, emission charges would not seem to be a proper approach for dealing with toxic or hazardous pollutants that *89*

must be controlled to specific levels.

There are a number of critical "pricing" subproblems. One is that, due to differences in meteorology, flow conditions, natural sources of pollutants, or concentrations of dischargers, geographic differences in ambient conditions make a uniform charge inappropriate. If the charge is set to solve the problems of areas needing much control, they will be excessive for areas needing little control and vice versa. A closely related problem is that unless a charge system differentiated among types of sources in setting charges, there could be substantial disruptive impacts. For example, charges needed to induce controls by steel mills could put nearby electroplaters out of business.

Thomas Tietenberg maintains that locally administered, spatially differentiated air pollutant emission charges offer a very real public option that would resolve these difficulties.[3] He, in fact, emphasizes that such charges are essential if the ambient air quality standards are to be achieved at minimum costs. Spatially differentiated charge systems are those in which the tax rate paid by an emitter is functionally related to the location of that emitter. Spatial differentiation could be built into an emission charge system either by increasing the number of geographically distinct taxing authorities or allowing each taxing jurisdiction to tax different emitters within its jurisdiction at different rates.

Another problem related to accurate "pricing" relates to changes over time. The method of determining the appropriate charge to levy on each kind of pollutant would be subject to frequent reassessment in a society with increasing population, affluence, and industrial capacity. If such decisions were not frequent, the environment would likely become progressively more polluted as more and more individuals, industries, and municipalities decided to pay discharge fees. Numerous practical questions would arise that differed only slightly from those that have arisen with regard to the permit system, with all of its attendant potential for negotiating and bargaining. Dischargers who in good faith had adjusted their emissions treatment to conform to a given level of charges and later saw the fee changed would complain bitterly, just as they now do under a shifting permit system. To avoid this reaction, taxes would have to be carefully set at the beginning, with a promise that they would remain unchanged for fixed periods of time. This raises the temptation to set the tax too high to ensure achieving the announced desired level of environmental quality. In highly concentrated industries, these costs could be passed on to the consumer, causing the burden of inefficiency to fall on the consumer and not the industry.

A final pricing-related problem involves the monitoring of emissions, because fee computation is so critically dependent on exact measurement of wastes. The accuracy of monitors is critical at all levels

of emissions where the computation of a charge is at stake, while in most regulatory approaches the accuracy of monitors is only critical at emission levels close to the standards.

Another effect, seen as a problem by some and as an advantage by others, is that an emission charge system would lead to a different pattern of control than the standards approach. Due to economies of scale of pollution control and longer amortization periods, larger and newer facilities would tend to have lower control costs per unit of pollution removed than do smaller and older plants. Hence, under a charge system, as compared to a standards approach, higher control costs would tend to be borne by larger and newer facilities while smaller or older ones would bear lower control costs.

All of these alleged advantages and problems have been discussed primarily in the theoretical literature. The key issue is how emission charge systems have worked out in practice.

Emission charges are in effect in France, the Netherlands, Hungary, the German Democratic Republic, and Czechoslovakia. In West Germany, the Water Act of 1976 stipulates that effluent charges will be implemented in 1981. Also, there are effluent charges in some provinces in Canada, for parts of some states in the United States, and in the Ruhr region of West Germany.

Actual effluent systems have three basic components: selecting the pollutants to assess and choosing how to add them up; estimating the waste discharge level of a polluter; and choosing the charge per unit of pollution over time.

In France, pollution charges vary in time and space and between basins, partly reflecting the quality of receiving water and the urgency of maintaining or restoring its quality. The charges are well below levels that provide an incentive to sharply decrease residuals discharge. In the Netherlands, sales in 1978 were between two and ten times higher than in the Seine-Normandy basin. In West Germany, polluters will be charged according to their reported discharge, with charges varying depending on the variability of discharge and the quality of water withdrawn.

In France, the charges have proved to be as subject to bargaining and as conditioned by considerations of political and administrative expediency as have standards, licenses, and other regulatory measures (such political realities aborted an attempt by the state legislature of Vermont to impose an emission charge system in the early 1970s). Perhaps because of this, charges have supplemented, not replaced, the traditional approaches. The charge system has, in fact, been used as part of a machinery of direct controls, serving as a method for spreading the burden of expenditure among polluters in ways that favor the major industrial interests, rather than as a means of efficiently achieving given levels of environmental quality. One study

of policy instruments for pollution control concluded that the instruments have not produced the results expected of them on the basis of their technical properties, nor have they brought about the profound changes in policymaking predicted by their advocates. It found that "the injection of new wine into old institutional bottles has not simplified, but actually complicated an already confused regulatory framework".[4]

Thus, it would appear that emission charges would have to be put into new wineskins. As phrased by three economists who have been leading advocates of emission charges, a "substantial political upheaval" would probably be required for acceptance of the "massive transfer of property rights" entailed by a system of charges.[5] Short of such radical change, along lines that have never been clearly spelled out, emission charges can be expected to be subject to pressures and institutional manipulations not dissimilar from those that have been shown to operate in the regulatory process.

Choosing the Best Approach

There is a developing consensus that a variety of approaches should be used simultaneously to cover the shortcomings inherent in each individual approach. In order to effectively manage an environmental quality problem through a variety of alternative strategies, criteria for the selection of a best strategy for any given situation must be developed. Suggested criteria for evaluating strategies follow:

1. Physical effects, or the degree that the physical method will: reduce the discharge of a residual from a specific source category; reduce a specific total discharge of the residual in the environmental quality management area; and change the relevant indicator(s) of environmental quality, which in turn may result in other physical effects such as decreased mortality or morbidity, decreased deterioration of materials, or increased fish biomass.

2. Economic effects, including: direct benefits or, where possible, the translation of the changes in physical effects into monetary value, such as reduced medical costs, reduced costs of cleaning and maintenance, or increased value of fish catch; the direct costs to the residuals dischargers—industrial plant, municipality, feedlot—of implementing the physical method in terms of capital, operating, and maintenance costs, or to the environmental quality management agency for implementing physical methods to reduce discharges or that directly affect assimilative capacity; administrative costs, both public and private, in terms of accounting and reporting, monitoring, analysis of samples, and supervision of operating personnel; and indirect economic effects, in terms of employment effects, changes in income

tax, changes in property taxes, increased cost of user goods, and dislocation of people.

A most important consideration with respect to both physical and economic effects is their distribution. Who benefits from improved environmental quality? Who pays and in what forms for the improvement? Distributional effects should be determined in relation to political jurisdictions and socioeconomic groups within the environmental quality management area, and the division between direct costs incurred within the area and those incurred external to the area; for example, the proportion of costs to be forthcoming from federal or state treasuries.

3. Flexibility in administration, or the administrative ease with which a strategy may be applied or removed, and the degree to which it remains effective under changed conditions. Consideration should be given to whether it can only be applied intermittently or continuously, as well as whether or not the strategy can be applied to selected activities—either within a category or among categories—or can only be applied to all activities generating the residual.

4. Simplicity in administration, or the procedural ease with which an incentive can be implemented. A major criticism of permit systems, for example, is the multiplicity and duplication of applications and approvals that must be obtained before an activity can operate.

5. Timing considerations related to the fact that strategies vary with respect to both the time required to put the physical method in place and into operation and the time required after it is in operation before the effect on environmental quality occurs. Timing is particularly important where adverse ambient conditions exist that need to be ameliorated as soon as possible. Timing is affected also by legal considerations. If new legislation must be enacted, implementation may take longer than if legal authority already exists. Public receptivity also affects timing. A strategy new to the public may require more time to implement than one that is not.

6. Political considerations would include at least six components. The first would be the policymaker's sense of his constituency's perception of the particular problem in relation to other environmental quality problems; for example, improved air quality vis-à-vis improved water quality. The second would be his constituency's perception of environmental quality management problems in relation to other social problems in the area, such as housing, transportation, and employment. A third would be the impact on intergovernmental relations, which should be considered vis-à-vis the strategy's effect on the normal way of doing the government's business. A fourth component would refer to the degree

to which an implementation incentive imposed at one level of government is consistent with those imposed at other levels of government. A fifth component would be public acceptance. Finally, the sixth component would relate to the degree of difficulty in obtaining legal authority for the institutional arrangement to impose the incentive. This includes such questions as: Does adequate authority to implement the strategy exist? Would existing legislation have to be changed to enable implementation, or would entirely new legislation have to be passed? Are questions of preemption, due process, or takings involved?

7. Intermedia effects should also be explicitly considered with regard to the quantities of other residuals generated and discharged into any of the environmental media. Three primary resource-use effects to be evaluated would include net energy required, net land required, and net consumptive use of water. An environmental quality management strategy may be energy intensive, or it may actually reduce total energy use in the area. The land required by a strategy to dispose of mixed solid residuals and sludge, for example, may be an important consideration in a densely urbanized area. The use of ponds, lagoons, and spray irrigation to reduce discharges may increase the net consumptive use of water in an area.[6]

Given that a variety of approaches must be used simultaneously, surely economic incentives such as the offset market, the bubble concept, or emission charges should be an integral part of any such package. Yet, such incentives must be regarded as piecemeal measures since they do not attack the root of the problem. Environmental protection and the reduction of social costs call for more fundamental methods of control.

Three types of measures are required. The first is strict public control over the use and disposal of toxic and other dangerous residuals. The second is the systematic development and promotion, under public auspices and perhaps in cooperation with industry, of technologies with a low ecological impact in order to reduce the degradation of the human environment by production and consumption activities. The systematic exploration of available alternative technologies and proposals, the promotion of research and development in these fields, and the formulation of an explicit science and technology policy directed toward low-impact technologies are prerequisites for the protection of the environment in the future. A third measure is aimed both at increasing the environment's capacity to assimilate residuals and developing new ways of recovering and reusing waste materials.

INTEGRATING PHYSICAL PRINCIPLES INTO ECONOMICS

Past Neglect

Though economics has always taught that there are three factors of production, sometime during the nineteenth century economists seemed to forget the importance of "land" (encompassing natural resources and the environment). Production functions in economic analysis consisted of labor and capital, which were brought together in the industrialization process in entirely new ways, enabling undreamed of production to take place, In this flush of excitement, the massive infusion of fuel and nonfuel minerals, which provided the basis for such a dynamic industrial thrust, went almost unnoticed since their supply was assured and their cost negligible relative to the other two factors. Only in recent years have economic principles textbooks begun inserting chapters on the environment or energy and, even then, these usually appear at the end along with other "miscellaneous" topics. Nor does the definitive study on sources of U.S. economic growth, *Accounting for United States Economic Growth 1929–1969,* even mention energy or natural resources as a contributing source. As E. F. Schumacher commented, it is inherent in the current methodology of economics to ignore man's dependence on the natural world.

Thus, economic theory today still studies the allocation of resources among competing ends, assuming that resources, personal tastes, and technology are given. Economists, concerned either with means of achieving high economic and productivity growth, equitable distribution, and low unemployment and inflation rates (or with explaining why such worthy goals are not achieved), pay little or no regard to evolutionary processes, to the dissipation of energy, or the depletion of resources. These aspects of the economic process are considered, if at all, as "externalities"; that is, as costs or benefits that are "external" to the theory of the firm or market.

In ignoring the Entropy Law, economists unwittingly have failed to realize that waste and pollution are not "external" to the economic process. Broadly, entropy measures the rate at which free or latent energy, available to do work, becomes bound energy no longer able to do work. The Entropy Law, the second law of thermodynamics, says simply that the entropy of energy systems increases constantly and irrevocably. This means that waste and pollution (i.e., bound energy unavailable to do work) increase inevitably in the flow of energy in any closed energy system. In ignoring the Entropy Law, economists have failed to realize a number of basic points: that in a productive process, entropy is just as inherent as productivity; that the product of the economic process is bound energy or waste; and that other things being the same, waste increases in greater proportion than the intensity of

economic activity.

The result is that economically efficient management is often quite at odds with ecologically sound management. The former (1) opts for the cheapest acceptable means of waste disposal, (2) uses the most cost-effective production processes, and (3) favors centralized sewage collection and processing, and dumping treated sewage into large tributaries and coastal oceans. The latter, to the contrary, (1) involves waste processing to produce usable by-products, (2) aims at closed industrial processes that minimize waste disposal demands on the environment, and (3) leads to recovery of nutrients and release of fresh water into surface water courses or ground water channels for further reuse.

Expanding the Theory and Policy

Economists can no longer ignore basic physical principles. They must acknowledge the nature of the interaction between the economy and the natural environment and integrate into their analytical systems the perspectives, central concepts, and theories that other disciplines have found relevant in clarifying the nature and causes of environmental disruption.

A necessary first step is to reverse the current theory in which the physical principles and conditions must accommodate the autonomous nonphysical conditions. In the new theory, physical parameters such as net energy, physical resource availability, a complex ecosystem and the laws of thermodynamics must come first; only then will it be asked how the nonphysical variables (such as technology, capital, preferences, and the distribution of wealth and income) can be brought into equilibrium with the complex biophysical system.

Alfred Marshall, one of the giants of economic thought, would have felt at home with this type of approach, for he frequently asserted that as economics became a mature science, biological analogies would displace mechanical analogies. Indeed, most of the leading economists, beginning with Adam Smith and continuing through Malthus and Marx to Keynes, acknowledged in their writings the significance of biological-economic analogies.

The new "physical economics" must recognize the basic distinction between conventional capital (buildings, equipment, and so forth) and biological capital (the ecosphere). The course of environmental deterioration shows that as conventional capital has accumulated since 1946, the value of the biological capital has declined. Environmental degradation represents a crucial, potentially fatal, hidden factor in the operation of the economic system. Thus, the effect of the operation of the economic system on the value of its biological capital needs to be taken into account in order to obtain a true estimate of the overall wealth-producing capability of the system.

Economics can no longer assume that resources are given or infinite. Economic policy alternatives must be evaluated as to how they relate to long-run ecological balance. This would reduce the risk of potentially disastrous disorder in the earth's systems of life support. Such a milestone in economic thought would lead to changes in the very definitions of output, income, wealth, productivity, cost, and profit.

In the 1980s, economic policies must be examined not only with respect to their impact upon such economic variables as investment, prices, employment, and income, but also on the rate of resource depletion and environmental deterioration.

FOOTNOTES TO CHAPTER 5

1. Alfred E. Kahn, "Environmental Values are Economic," *Challenge,* May–June 1979, p. 67.

2. The four principal articles drawn upon throughout this section are "Giandomeniao Majone, "Choice among Policy Instruments for Pollution Control," *Policy Analysis,* Fall 1976; Lettie McSpadden Wenner, "Pollution Control: Implementation Alternatives," *Policy Analysis,* Winter 1978; Russell E. Train, "Emission Charges and other Economic Approaches to Environmental Programs," *Tax Notes,* February 23, 1977; James Booth and Zena Cook, *An Exploration of Regulatory Incentives for Innovation: Six Case Studies,* Public Interest Economics Center paper for National Bureau of Standards, January 18, 1979.

3. T. H. Tietenberg, "Spatially Differentiated Air Pollutant Emission Charges: An Economic and Legal Analysis," *Land Economics,* August 1978.

4. Majone, op cit, p. 589.

5. A. Myrick Freeman, Robert Haveman, and Allen V. Kneese, *Economics of Environmental Policy,* p. 170.

6. Blair T. Bower, Charles N. Ehler, and Allen V. Kneese, "Incentives for Managing the Environment," *Environmental Science and Technology,* March 1977, pp. 253–54.

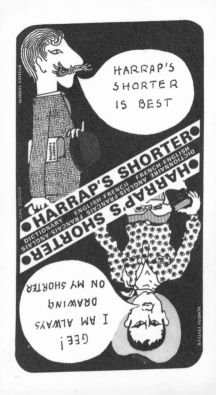

H A R R A P ' S
S H O R T E R

DICTIONARY

ANGLAIS-FRANÇAIS
FRANÇAIS-ANGLAIS

LE PLUS COMPLET
LE PLUS MODERNE
LE PLUS CLASSIQUE
DES
DICTIONNAIRES

1 506 pages. 97 000 articles. Format 23,5 × 16,2. Reliure toile sous jaquette illustrée . . . . 45 F

BORDAS

EN VENTE CHEZ TOUS LES LIBRAIRES